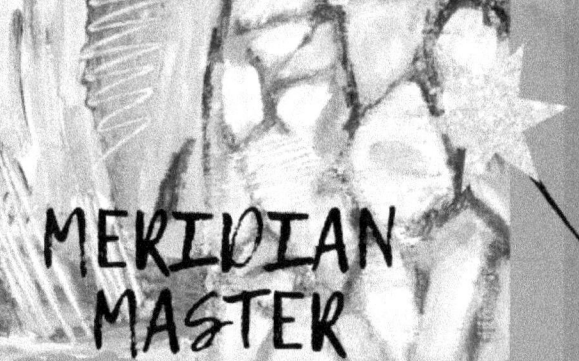

MERIDIAN MASTER

A Journey Through the Twelve Major Pathways

Mei Lin Zhang

Table of Contents

Meridian Master A Journey Through the Twelve Major Pathways 1

Introduction to the Twelve Major Meridians 2

The Concept of Meridians 5

The Importance of Meridians in Traditional Chinese Medicine 7

The Lung Meridian 9

Anatomy and Pathway 11

Acupressure Points and Functions 13

The Large Intestine Meridian 15

The Stomach Meridian 17

The Spleen Meridian 19

The Heart Meridian 21

The Small Intestine Meridian 23

The Bladder Meridian 25

The Kidney Meridian 27

The Pericardium Meridian 29

The Triple Warmer Meridian 31

The Gallbladder Meridian 33

The Liver Meridian 35

Yin and Yang Meridians 37

The Concept of Yin and Yang 39

The Relationship Between Yin and Yang Meridians 42

The Five Elements and Meridians 44

Introduction to the Five Elements 47

The Relationship Between Meridians and the Five Elements 49

The Meridian Clock 52

The Concept of the Meridian Clock 54

How to Use the Meridian Clock for Optimal Health 57

Meridian Diagnosis and Assessment 60

The Importance of Meridian Diagnosis 62

Methods for Assessing Meridian Health 64

Acupressure Techniques 67

Introduction to Acupressure 70

How to Apply Acupressure on Meridian Points 73

Acupuncture and Meridians 76

Introduction to Acupuncture 79

How Acupuncture Works with the Meridian System 82

Moxibustion and Meridians 84

Introduction to Moxibustion 86

The Benefits of Moxibustion on Meridian Health 89

Cupping Therapy and Meridians 92

Introduction to Cupping Therapy	94
How Cupping Therapy Affects the Meridian System	96
Qigong and Meridian Exercises	99
Introduction to Qigong	101
Meridian Exercises for Health and Balance	103
Meridian Meditation Techniques	106
The Importance of Meditation	109
Meridian-Based Meditation Practices	111
The Role of Nutrition in Meridian Health	114
The Importance of a Balanced Diet	116
Foods That Support Meridian Health	119
Maintaining Meridian Balance for Optimal Health	122
The Importance of Regular Meridian Care	124
Lifestyle Tips for Supporting Meridian Health	126
Emotional and Mental Health and the Meridians	128
The Connection Between Emotions and Meridian Health	130
Techniques for Balancing Emotions Through Meridian Work	132
Meridian Massage Techniques	135
Introduction to Meridian Massage	137
How to Perform a Meridian Massage	139
Essential Oils and the Meridians	141

Introduction to Essential Oils 143

Using Essential Oils for Meridian Health... 145

The Connection Between Meridians and Chakras 147

The Chakra System Explained 149

The Relationship Between Meridians and Chakras 151

Common Meridian Imbalances and Their Symptoms........................ 153

Recognizing Meridian Imbalances... 156

Addressing Imbalances Through Meridian Work................................ 159

The Role of Herbs in Meridian Health 161

Introduction to Herbal Medicine 163

Herbs for Supporting Meridian Health 165

The Connection Between Meridians and the Immune System 167

The Importance of a Healthy Immune System 169

How Meridian Work Supports Immune Health................................. 171

Meridian Health and Sleep... 174

The Importance of Quality Sleep 176

How Meridian Work Can Improve Sleep... 179

Meridian Health and Aging 182

The Aging Process and Its Effects on Meridians................................. 184

How to Support Meridian Health as We Age 186

The Role of Meridians in Pain Management 188

Understanding Chronic Pain 191

How Meridian Work Can Help Manage Pain 194

Integrating Meridian Work into Daily Life 196

Tips for Incorporating Meridian Practices 199

Creating a Personalized Meridian Routine 201

The Future of Meridian Research 203

Current Research and Findings 206

The Potential for Future Developments in Meridian Health 208

The Importance of Meridian Health 210

Embracing a Meridian-Based Lifestyle for Optimal Well-being 212

Have Questions / Comments? 215

Get Another Book Free 216

Created by Xspurts.com[1]

All rights reserved.

Copyright © 2005 onwards .

By reading this book, you agree to the below Terms and Conditions.

Xspurts.com[2] retains all rights to these products.

No part of this book may be reproduced in any form, by photostat, microfilm, xerography, or any other means, or incorporated into any information retrieval system, electronic or mechanical, without the written permission of Xspurts.com[3]; exceptions are made for brief excerpts used in published reviews.

This publication is designed to provide accurate and authoritative information with regard to the subject matter covered, however is for entertainment purposes only. It is sold with the understanding that the publisher is not engaged in rendering legal, accounting, health, relationship or other professional / personal advice. If legal advice or other expert assistance is required, the services of a competent professional should be sought.

First Printed 2023.

ISBN:

DIGITAL VERSION: 978-1-77684-935-2

PHYSICAL VERSION: 978-1-77684-868-3

- A New Zealand Designed Product

Get A Free Book At: go.xspurts.com/free-book-offer[4]

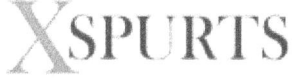

---

1. https://Xspurts.com
2. https://Xspurts.com
3. https://Xspurts.com
4. https://go.xspurts.com/free-book-offer
5. https://xspurts.com/

Introduction to the Twelve Major Meridians

The concept of meridians is an integral part of Traditional Chinese Medicine (TCM). Meridians are believed to be channels in the body through which vital energy or Qi flows. The flow of Qi is essential for maintaining physical, emotional, and spiritual balance. The meridian system consists of twelve major meridians and eight extraordinary meridians. Below we will focus on the twelve major meridians.

The twelve major meridians are divided into six pairs, with each pair corresponding to one of the five elements: wood, fire, earth, metal, and water. The five elements represent the basic substances and processes in nature and are believed to be closely related to human health.

The first pair of meridians is the Lung and Large Intestine meridians, corresponding to the metal element. The Lung meridian begins in the chest and runs down the arm to the thumb. It is associated with respiration and the immune system. The Large Intestine meridian starts at the index finger and runs up the arm to the head. It is responsible for the elimination of waste and toxins from the body.

The second pair is the Stomach and Spleen meridians, corresponding to the earth element. The Stomach meridian starts at the head and runs down the body to the foot. It is responsible for digestion and nourishment. The Spleen meridian runs from the foot to the chest and is associated with the production of Qi and blood.

The third pair is the Heart and Small Intestine meridians, corresponding to the fire element. The Heart meridian begins in the chest and runs down the arm to the pinky finger. It is responsible for circulation and emotional well-being. The Small Intestine meridian runs up the arm to the head and is associated with the absorption and distribution of nutrients.

The fourth pair is the Bladder and Kidney meridians, corresponding to the water element. The Bladder meridian starts at the head and runs down the back of the body to the foot. It is responsible for the elimination of waste and maintaining water balance in the body. The Kidney meridian runs up the inside of the leg to the chest and is associated with the production of hormones and the regulation of fluid balance.

The fifth pair is the Pericardium and Triple Burner meridians, corresponding to the fire element. The Pericardium meridian begins in the chest and runs down the arm to the middle finger. It is associated with the heart and emotional well-being. The Triple Burner meridian runs up the arm to the head and is responsible for regulating the body's temperature and fluids.

The sixth pair is the Gallbladder and Liver meridians, corresponding to the wood element. The Gallbladder meridian starts at the head and runs down the side of the body to the foot. It is responsible for the digestion and metabolism of fats. The Liver meridian runs up the inside of the leg to the chest and is associated with detoxification and the regulation of Qi.

Each of the twelve major meridians has specific points along its path that can be stimulated by acupuncture or acupressure to promote the flow of Qi and balance the body's energy. These points are known as acupoints and are located at specific anatomical locations.

In TCM, the twelve major meridians are also associated with different emotions and states of mind. For example, the Lung meridian is associated with grief, the Stomach meridian with worry, the Heart meridian with joy, and the Liver meridian with anger. By understanding these associations, TCM practitioners can use acupuncture and other techniques to help balance emotions and promote overall well-being.

The Concept of Meridians

The concept of meridians is a central part of Traditional Chinese Medicine (TCM) and has been used for thousands of years to promote health and well-being. According to TCM, meridians are channels in the body through which vital energy or Qi flows. The flow of Qi is essential for maintaining physical, emotional, and spiritual balance.

The meridian system consists of twelve major meridians and eight extraordinary meridians. The twelve major meridians are the Lung, Large Intestine, Stomach, Spleen, Heart, Small Intestine, Bladder, Kidney, Pericardium, Triple Burner, Gallbladder, and Liver meridians. Each of these meridians has a specific path in the body and is associated with different organs, functions, and emotions.

The eight extraordinary meridians are considered to be deeper and more complex than the twelve major meridians. They are believed to play a significant role in regulating the body's energy and maintaining overall health. These meridians are the Governor Vessel, Conception Vessel, Belt Vessel, Yin Linking Vessel, Yang Linking Vessel, Yin Heel Vessel, Yang Heel Vessel, and Penetrating Vessel.

The concept of meridians is based on the principles of Yin and Yang, which are the two opposing forces in nature. Yin represents the feminine, dark, and passive energy, while Yang represents the masculine, light, and active energy. According to TCM, the body is in a state of balance when Yin and Yang are in harmony. Imbalances in Yin and Yang can lead to illness, pain, and emotional distress.

The flow of Qi along the meridians is influenced by many factors, including emotions, diet, lifestyle, and environmental factors. When Qi is blocked or stagnant, it can lead to physical and emotional symptoms. TCM practitioners use various techniques, such as acupuncture, acupressure, herbal medicine, and dietary therapy, to promote the flow of Qi and restore balance to the body.

Acupuncture is one of the most well-known techniques used in TCM to stimulate the flow of Qi along the meridians. Acupuncture involves inserting fine needles into specific acupoints along the meridians to stimulate the flow of Qi and promote healing. Acupressure is a similar technique that involves applying pressure to specific acupoints using the fingers, hands, or other tools.

Herbal medicine is another common practice in TCM that involves using plants and herbs to promote healing and balance. Different herbs are believed to have specific effects on the body and can be combined in formulas to treat specific conditions. Dietary therapy is also an important aspect of TCM and involves using food as medicine to promote health and prevent illness.

The concept of meridians is not widely accepted in Western medicine, and there is limited scientific evidence to support its effectiveness. However, many people have found TCM practices, such as acupuncture and herbal medicine, to be helpful in treating various conditions and promoting overall well-being.

The Importance of Meridians in Traditional Chinese Medicine

Meridians are a central concept in Traditional Chinese Medicine (TCM) and play an essential role in maintaining physical, emotional, and spiritual balance. Meridians are believed to be channels in the body through which vital energy or Qi flows. The flow of Qi along these meridians is crucial for maintaining health and preventing illness.

In TCM, there are twelve major meridians that run throughout the body, each associated with different organs, functions, and emotions. These twelve meridians are the Lung, Large Intestine, Stomach, Spleen, Heart, Small Intestine, Bladder, Kidney, Pericardium, Triple Burner, Gallbladder, and Liver meridians. Each of these meridians has specific acupoints along its path that can be stimulated to promote the flow of Qi and restore balance to the body.

The importance of meridians in TCM lies in their role in regulating the flow of Qi. Qi is considered the vital energy that animates the body and provides the power for all life processes. When Qi flows smoothly along the meridians, the body is in a state of balance, and health is maintained. However, when the flow of Qi is blocked or stagnant, it can lead to physical and emotional symptoms and ultimately result in illness.

The twelve major meridians are associated with different organs and functions in the body. For example, the Lung meridian is associated with respiration and the immune system, while the Large Intestine meridian is responsible for the elimination of waste and toxins from the body. The Stomach meridian is associated with digestion and nourishment, while the Spleen meridian is responsible for the production of Qi and blood.

In TCM, emotions are also believed to be closely connected to the meridians. Each of the twelve major meridians is associated with different emotions, and imbalances in these emotions can lead to disruptions in the flow of Qi along the meridians. For example, the Lung meridian is associated with grief, the Stomach meridian with worry, and the Liver meridian with anger. By understanding these associations, TCM practitioners can use acupuncture and other techniques to help balance emotions and promote overall well-being.

Acupuncture is one of the most well-known techniques used in TCM to stimulate the flow of Qi along the meridians. Acupuncture involves inserting fine needles into specific acupoints along the meridians to stimulate the flow of Qi and promote healing. Acupressure is a similar technique that involves applying pressure to specific acupoints using the fingers, hands, or other tools.

Herbal medicine is another important aspect of TCM that can be used to support the flow of Qi along the meridians. Different herbs are believed to have specific effects on the body and can be combined in formulas to treat specific conditions. For example, herbs that are believed to support the Lung meridian include mulberry leaf, apricot kernel, and lily bulb.

Dietary therapy is also an important aspect of TCM and involves using food as medicine to promote health and prevent illness. Different foods are believed to have specific effects on the body and can be used to support the flow of Qi along the meridians. For example, foods that are believed to support the Spleen meridian include rice, barley, and sweet potato.

The Lung Meridian

The Lung meridian is one of the twelve major meridians in Traditional Chinese Medicine (TCM) and is associated with the Lung organ and the respiratory system. The Lung meridian runs from the chest to the thumb and is responsible for the regulation of Qi and the immune system.

In TCM, the Lung is considered the organ that receives and distributes Qi from the outside world, making it the first line of defense against external pathogens. The Lung meridian is believed to regulate the flow of Qi in the body and maintain the balance between the interior and exterior environment.

The Lung meridian starts in the chest and runs down the arm, ending at the thumb. Along its path, there are various acupoints that can be stimulated to promote the flow of Qi and restore balance to the body. Some of the key acupoints along the Lung meridian include the Lung 1, Lung 5, and Lung

Lung 1 is located on the upper chest, close to the shoulder. It is believed to be the starting point of the Lung meridian and is often used to treat respiratory issues such as asthma and coughs. Stimulating this acupoint is also believed to promote the flow of Qi and help reduce anxiety and tension.

Lung 5 is located on the forearm, near the wrist. It is associated with the regulation of Qi and is often used to treat respiratory issues such as bronchitis and pneumonia. Stimulating this acupoint is also believed to help alleviate pain and reduce swelling in the arm and wrist.

Lung 7 is located on the wrist, on the thumb side of the hand. It is believed to be a key acupoint for the regulation of Qi and the immune system. Stimulating this acupoint is also believed to help alleviate coughs, reduce stress and anxiety, and improve overall well-being.

In TCM, the Lung meridian is also associated with specific emotions, such as grief and sadness. Imbalances in these emotions can lead to disruptions in the flow of Qi along the Lung meridian and ultimately result in physical symptoms such as shortness of breath and coughing.

TCM practitioners use various techniques, such as acupuncture and acupressure, to stimulate the flow of Qi along the Lung meridian and restore balance to the body. Acupuncture involves the insertion of fine needles into specific acupoints along the meridian to promote the flow of Qi and restore balance. Acupressure is a similar technique that involves applying pressure to specific acupoints using the fingers, hands, or other tools.

In addition to acupuncture and acupressure, dietary therapy is also an essential aspect of TCM that can be used to support the Lung meridian. Foods that are believed to support the Lung meridian include pears, white rice, and almonds. These foods are believed to have a cooling and moistening effect on the body, which can help alleviate dryness and promote the flow of Qi.

Anatomy and Pathway

The twelve major meridians in Traditional Chinese Medicine (TCM) are channels in the body through which vital energy or Qi flows. Each meridian has a specific pathway and is associated with different organs, functions, and emotions. Understanding the anatomy and pathway of these meridians is essential for TCM practitioners to diagnose and treat various conditions.

The Lung meridian, for example, starts in the chest and runs down the arm, ending at the thumb. The Large Intestine meridian starts at the index finger and runs up the arm, through the shoulder and neck, and ends at the nose. The Stomach meridian starts at the second toe and runs up the leg, through the abdomen and chest, and ends at the lower lip.

The pathways of the meridians are not limited to the surface of the body but also extend deep into the body, connecting various organs and tissues. The meridians are interconnected and form a complex network throughout the body, regulating the flow of Qi and maintaining overall health and well-being.

In TCM, each meridian is associated with specific functions and emotions. For example, the Lung meridian is associated with respiration and the immune system, as well as the emotions of grief and sadness. The Large Intestine meridian is associated with elimination and the emotions of guilt and shame. The Stomach meridian is associated with digestion and nourishment, as well as the emotions of worry and overthinking.

The meridians are also believed to have an impact on the flow of blood and other bodily fluids. According to TCM, when the flow of Qi is disrupted, it can lead to imbalances in the flow of blood and other bodily fluids, resulting in physical symptoms such as pain, swelling, and inflammation.

In TCM, the anatomy and pathway of the meridians are crucial for the diagnosis and treatment of various conditions. TCM practitioners use various techniques, such as pulse diagnosis, tongue diagnosis, and palpation of the acupoints along the meridians, to identify imbalances in the flow of Qi and diagnose specific conditions.

Acupuncture is one of the most well-known techniques used in TCM to stimulate the flow of Qi along the meridians. Acupuncture involves inserting fine needles into specific acupoints along the meridians to stimulate the flow of Qi and promote healing. Each acupoint is believed to have specific effects on the body and can be used to treat specific conditions.

Herbal medicine is another common practice in TCM that involves using plants and herbs to promote healing and balance. Different herbs are believed to have specific effects on the body and can be combined in formulas to treat specific conditions. For example, herbs that are believed to support the Lung meridian include mulberry leaf, apricot kernel, and lily bulb.

Dietary therapy is also an essential aspect of TCM and involves using food as medicine to promote health and prevent illness. Different foods are believed to have specific effects on the body and can be used to support the flow of Qi along the meridians. For example, foods that are believed to support the Spleen meridian include rice, barley, and sweet potato.

Acupressure Points and Functions

Acupressure is a healing technique in Traditional Chinese Medicine (TCM) that involves applying pressure to specific points on the body to stimulate the flow of Qi and promote healing. These points, also known as acupoints, are located along the twelve major meridians in the body and have specific functions and benefits.

The Lung meridian, for example, has several acupoints that can be used to promote respiratory health and reduce stress and anxiety. Lung 1, located on the upper chest, is often used to treat respiratory issues such as asthma and coughs. Stimulating this acupoint is also believed to promote the flow of Qi and help reduce anxiety and tension. Lung 7, located on the wrist, is believed to be a key acupoint for the regulation of Qi and the immune system. Stimulating this acupoint is also believed to help alleviate coughs, reduce stress and anxiety, and improve overall well-being.

The Large Intestine meridian has several acupoints that can be used to treat digestive issues and promote detoxification. Large Intestine 4, located between the thumb and index finger, is often used to treat headaches, toothaches, and digestive issues such as constipation and diarrhea. Stimulating this acupoint is also believed to promote the flow of Qi and help detoxify the body.

The Stomach meridian has several acupoints that can be used to promote digestion and reduce nausea and vomiting. Stomach 36, located on the lower leg, is often used to treat digestive issues such as bloating, gas, and indigestion. Stimulating this acupoint is also believed to help reduce stress and anxiety and promote overall well-being.

The Spleen meridian has several acupoints that can be used to support the production of Qi and blood and promote overall health and vitality. Spleen 6, located on the lower leg, is often used to treat menstrual issues such as cramps and irregular periods. Stimulating this acupoint is also believed to help support digestion, promote the production of Qi and blood, and reduce stress and anxiety.

The Heart meridian has several acupoints that can be used to promote heart health and reduce anxiety and depression. Heart 7, located on the wrist, is often used to treat insomnia, anxiety, and depression. Stimulating this acupoint is also believed to promote heart health and reduce stress and tension.

The Small Intestine meridian has several acupoints that can be used to treat digestive issues and promote overall health and well-being. Small Intestine 3, located on the outer edge of the hand, is often used to treat headaches and digestive issues such as bloating and gas. Stimulating this acupoint is also believed to promote the flow of Qi and help reduce stress and tension.

The Bladder meridian has several acupoints that can be used to promote urinary health and reduce back pain. Bladder 23, located on the lower back, is often used to treat urinary issues such as frequent urination and bladder infections. Stimulating this acupoint is also believed to help reduce back pain and promote overall well-being.

The Kidney meridian has several acupoints that can be used to support kidney health and promote overall well-being. Kidney 1, located on the sole of the foot, is often used to treat urinary issues such as incontinence and frequent urination. Stimulating this acupoint is also believed to help promote the flow of Qi and blood and support kidney health.

The Large Intestine Meridian

The Large Intestine meridian is one of the twelve major meridians in Traditional Chinese Medicine (TCM) and is associated with the Large Intestine organ and the elimination system. The Large Intestine meridian starts at the index finger and runs up the arm, through the shoulder and neck, and ends at the nose. Along its pathway, there are various acupoints that can be stimulated to promote the flow of Qi and restore balance to the body.

In TCM, the Large Intestine is considered the organ that eliminates waste and toxins from the body. The Large Intestine meridian is believed to regulate the flow of Qi in the body and maintain the balance between the interior and exterior environment. Stimulating the acupoints along the Large Intestine meridian can help promote the flow of Qi and restore balance to the body.

Large Intestine 4 is one of the key acupoints along the Large Intestine meridian and is located between the thumb and index finger. It is often used to treat headaches, toothaches, and digestive issues such as constipation and diarrhea. Stimulating this acupoint is also believed to promote the flow of Qi and help detoxify the body.

Another important acupoint along the Large Intestine meridian is Large Intestine 11, located at the outer end of the elbow crease. This acupoint is often used to treat joint pain and inflammation, as well as digestive issues such as constipation and diarrhea. Stimulating this acupoint is also believed to promote the flow of Qi and help reduce stress and tension in the body.

Large Intestine 20 is located at the side of the nostrils and is believed to be a key acupoint for the respiratory system. Stimulating this acupoint is often used to treat nasal congestion, sinusitis, and allergies. It is also believed to promote the flow of Qi and help reduce stress and tension in the body.

In addition to acupuncture and acupressure, dietary therapy is also an essential aspect of TCM that can be used to support the Large Intestine meridian. Foods that are believed to support the Large Intestine meridian include pears, apples, and radishes. These foods are believed to have a cooling and cleansing effect on the body, which can help promote the elimination of waste and toxins.

In TCM, the Large Intestine meridian is also associated with specific emotions, such as guilt and shame. Imbalances in these emotions can lead to disruptions in the flow of Qi along the Large Intestine meridian and ultimately result in physical symptoms such as constipation and diarrhea.

TCM practitioners use various techniques, such as acupuncture and acupressure, to stimulate the flow of Qi along the Large Intestine meridian and restore balance to the body. Acupuncture involves the insertion of fine needles into specific acupoints along the meridian to promote the flow of Qi and restore balance. Acupressure is a similar technique that involves applying pressure to specific acupoints using the fingers, hands, or other tools.

The Stomach Meridian

The Stomach meridian is one of the twelve major meridians in Traditional Chinese Medicine (TCM) and is associated with the Stomach organ and the digestive system. The Stomach meridian starts at the second toe and runs up the leg, through the abdomen and chest, and ends at the lower lip. Along its pathway, there are various acupoints that can be stimulated to promote the flow of Qi and restore balance to the body.

In TCM, the Stomach is considered the organ responsible for the digestion and absorption of food. The Stomach meridian is believed to regulate the flow of Qi in the body and maintain the balance between the interior and exterior environment. Stimulating the acupoints along the Stomach meridian can help promote the flow of Qi and restore balance to the body.

Stomach 36 is one of the key acupoints along the Stomach meridian and is located on the lower leg, about four finger widths below the knee. It is often used to treat digestive issues such as bloating, gas, and indigestion. Stimulating this acupoint is also believed to help reduce stress and anxiety and promote overall well-being.

Another important acupoint along the Stomach meridian is Stomach 42, located on the foot between the second and third toe. This acupoint is often used to treat digestive issues such as nausea and vomiting. Stimulating this acupoint is also believed to promote the flow of Qi and help reduce stress and tension in the body.

Stomach 44 is located on the upper lip and is believed to be a key acupoint for the digestive system. Stimulating this acupoint is often used to treat digestive issues such as bloating and indigestion. It is also believed to promote the flow of Qi and help reduce stress and tension in the body.

In addition to acupuncture and acupressure, dietary therapy is also an essential aspect of TCM that can be used to support the Stomach meridian. Foods that are believed to support the Stomach meridian include rice, barley, and sweet potato. These foods are believed to have a nourishing and strengthening effect on the body, which can help support the digestion and absorption of food.

In TCM, the Stomach meridian is also associated with specific emotions, such as worry and overthinking. Imbalances in these emotions can lead to disruptions in the flow of Qi along the Stomach meridian and ultimately result in physical symptoms such as digestive issues.

TCM practitioners use various techniques, such as acupuncture and acupressure, to stimulate the flow of Qi along the Stomach meridian and restore balance to the body. Acupuncture involves the insertion of fine needles into specific acupoints along the meridian to promote the flow of Qi and restore balance. Acupressure is a similar technique that involves applying pressure to specific acupoints using the fingers, hands, or other tools.

The Spleen Meridian

The Spleen meridian is one of the twelve major meridians in Traditional Chinese Medicine (TCM) and is associated with the Spleen organ and the digestive system. The Spleen meridian starts at the big toe and runs up the leg, through the abdomen and chest, and ends at the ribcage. Along its pathway, there are various acupoints that can be stimulated to promote the flow of Qi and restore balance to the body.

In TCM, the Spleen is considered the organ responsible for the transformation and transportation of food and fluids in the body. The Spleen meridian is believed to regulate the flow of Qi in the body and maintain the balance between the interior and exterior environment. Stimulating the acupoints along the Spleen meridian can help promote the flow of Qi and restore balance to the body.

Spleen 6 is one of the key acupoints along the Spleen meridian and is located on the lower leg, about three finger widths above the ankle. It is often used to treat menstrual issues such as cramps and irregular periods. Stimulating this acupoint is also believed to help support digestion, promote the production of Qi and blood, and reduce stress and anxiety.

Another important acupoint along the Spleen meridian is Spleen 9, located on the lower leg, just above the anklebone. This acupoint is often used to treat digestive issues such as bloating and gas. Stimulating this acupoint is also believed to promote the flow of Qi and help reduce stress and tension in the body.

Spleen 21 is located on the side of the ribcage and is believed to be a key acupoint for the reproductive system. Stimulating this acupoint is often used to treat menstrual issues such as cramps and irregular periods. It is also believed to promote the flow of Qi and help reduce stress and tension in the body.

In addition to acupuncture and acupressure, dietary therapy is also an essential aspect of TCM that can be used to support the Spleen meridian. Foods that are believed to support the Spleen meridian include rice, barley, and pumpkin. These foods are believed to have a nourishing and strengthening effect on the body, which can help support the digestion and absorption of food.

In TCM, the Spleen meridian is also associated with specific emotions, such as worry and overthinking. Imbalances in these emotions can lead to disruptions in the flow of Qi along the Spleen meridian and ultimately result in physical symptoms such as digestive issues and fatigue.

TCM practitioners use various techniques, such as acupuncture and acupressure, to stimulate the flow of Qi along the Spleen meridian and restore balance to the body. Acupuncture involves the insertion of fine needles into specific acupoints along the meridian to promote the flow of Qi and restore balance. Acupressure is a similar technique that involves applying pressure to specific acupoints using the fingers, hands, or other tools.

The Heart Meridian

The Heart meridian is one of the twelve major meridians in Traditional Chinese Medicine (TCM) and is associated with the Heart organ and the circulatory system. The Heart meridian starts at the armpit and runs down the arm, through the wrist and hand, and ends at the tip of the little finger. Along its pathway, there are various acupoints that can be stimulated to promote the flow of Qi and restore balance to the body.

In TCM, the Heart is considered the organ responsible for the circulation of blood and the regulation of emotions. The Heart meridian is believed to regulate the flow of Qi in the body and maintain the balance between the interior and exterior environment. Stimulating the acupoints along the Heart meridian can help promote the flow of Qi and restore balance to the body.

Heart 7 is one of the key acupoints along the Heart meridian and is located on the wrist, at the crease of the hand. It is often used to treat insomnia and anxiety. Stimulating this acupoint is also believed to help regulate the heartbeat and promote the circulation of Qi and blood.

Another important acupoint along the Heart meridian is Heart 5, located on the inner wrist, in line with the little finger. This acupoint is often used to treat heart-related issues such as palpitations and chest pain. Stimulating this acupoint is also believed to promote the flow of Qi and help reduce stress and tension in the body.

Heart 1 is located on the armpit and is believed to be a key acupoint for the Heart meridian. Stimulating this acupoint is often used to treat heart-related issues such as chest pain and palpitations. It is also believed to promote the flow of Qi and help reduce stress and tension in the body.

In addition to acupuncture and acupressure, dietary therapy is also an essential aspect of TCM that can be used to support the Heart meridian. Foods that are believed to support the Heart meridian include cherries, red beans, and beets. These foods are believed to have a nourishing and strengthening effect on the body, which can help support the circulation of blood and the regulation of emotions.

In TCM, the Heart meridian is also associated with specific emotions, such as joy and anxiety. Imbalances in these emotions can lead to disruptions in the flow of Qi along the Heart meridian and ultimately result in physical symptoms such as chest pain and palpitations.

TCM practitioners use various techniques, such as acupuncture and acupressure, to stimulate the flow of Qi along the Heart meridian and restore balance to the body. Acupuncture involves the insertion of fine needles into specific acupoints along the meridian to promote the flow of Qi and restore balance. Acupressure is a similar technique that involves applying pressure to specific acupoints using the fingers, hands, or other tools.

The Small Intestine Meridian

The Small Intestine meridian is one of the twelve major meridians in Traditional Chinese Medicine (TCM) and is associated with the Small Intestine organ and the digestive system. The Small Intestine meridian starts at the outer tip of the little finger and runs up the arm, through the shoulder and neck, and ends at the ear. Along its pathway, there are various acupoints that can be stimulated to promote the flow of Qi and restore balance to the body.

In TCM, the Small Intestine is considered the organ responsible for separating the pure and impure substances in the body. The Small Intestine meridian is believed to regulate the flow of Qi in the body and maintain the balance between the interior and exterior environment. Stimulating the acupoints along the Small Intestine meridian can help promote the flow of Qi and restore balance to the body.

Small Intestine 3 is one of the key acupoints along the Small Intestine meridian and is located on the hand, at the outer edge of the fist. It is often used to treat shoulder and neck pain. Stimulating this acupoint is also believed to help promote the flow of Qi and blood, and reduce stress and tension in the body.

Another important acupoint along the Small Intestine meridian is Small Intestine 6, located on the wrist, in line with the little finger. This acupoint is often used to treat digestive issues such as bloating and diarrhea. Stimulating this acupoint is also believed to promote the flow of Qi and help reduce stress and tension in the body.

Small Intestine 19 is located in front of the ear and is believed to be a key acupoint for the Small Intestine meridian. Stimulating this acupoint is often used to treat ear-related issues such as tinnitus and deafness. It is also believed to promote the flow of Qi and help reduce stress and tension in the body.

In addition to acupuncture and acupressure, dietary therapy is also an essential aspect of TCM that can be used to support the Small Intestine meridian. Foods that are believed to support the Small Intestine meridian include ginger, green onions, and coriander. These foods are believed to have a warming and dispersing effect on the body, which can help support the digestion and absorption of food.

In TCM, the Small Intestine meridian is also associated with specific emotions, such as anxiety and nervousness. Imbalances in these emotions can lead to disruptions in the flow of Qi along the Small Intestine meridian and ultimately result in physical symptoms such as digestive issues and ear-related issues.

TCM practitioners use various techniques, such as acupuncture and acupressure, to stimulate the flow of Qi along the Small Intestine meridian and restore balance to the body. Acupuncture involves the insertion of fine needles into specific acupoints along the meridian to promote the flow of Qi and restore balance. Acupressure is a similar technique that involves applying pressure to specific acupoints using the fingers, hands, or other tools.

The Bladder Meridian

The Bladder meridian is one of the twelve major meridians in Traditional Chinese Medicine (TCM) and is associated with the Bladder organ and the urinary system. The Bladder meridian starts at the inner corner of the eye and runs down the back, through the legs and feet, and ends at the little toe. Along its pathway, there are various acupoints that can be stimulated to promote the flow of Qi and restore balance to the body.

In TCM, the Bladder is considered the organ responsible for the storage and elimination of urine. The Bladder meridian is believed to regulate the flow of Qi in the body and maintain the balance between the interior and exterior environment. Stimulating the acupoints along the Bladder meridian can help promote the flow of Qi and restore balance to the body.

Bladder 23 is one of the key acupoints along the Bladder meridian and is located on the lower back, on either side of the spine. It is often used to treat lower back pain and urinary issues. Stimulating this acupoint is also believed to help strengthen the kidneys and promote the flow of Qi and blood.

Another important acupoint along the Bladder meridian is Bladder 40, located on the back of the leg, just below the knee. This acupoint is often used to treat knee pain and stiffness. Stimulating this acupoint is also believed to promote the flow of Qi and help reduce stress and tension in the body.

Bladder 67 is located on the outer corner of the little toenail and is believed to be a key acupoint for the Bladder meridian. Stimulating this acupoint is often used to help turn a breech baby during pregnancy. It is also believed to promote the flow of Qi and help reduce stress and tension in the body.

In addition to acupuncture and acupressure, dietary therapy is also an essential aspect of TCM that can be used to support the Bladder meridian. Foods that are believed to support the Bladder meridian include watermelon, celery, and dandelion greens. These foods are believed to have a diuretic and cooling effect on the body, which can help support the urinary system.

In TCM, the Bladder meridian is also associated with specific emotions, such as fear and anxiety. Imbalances in these emotions can lead to disruptions in the flow of Qi along the Bladder meridian and ultimately result in physical symptoms such as lower back pain and urinary issues.

TCM practitioners use various techniques, such as acupuncture and acupressure, to stimulate the flow of Qi along the Bladder meridian and restore balance to the body. Acupuncture involves the insertion of fine needles into specific acupoints along the meridian to promote the flow of Qi and restore balance. Acupressure is a similar technique that involves applying pressure to specific acupoints using the fingers, hands, or other tools.

The Kidney Meridian

The Kidney meridian is one of the twelve major meridians in Traditional Chinese Medicine (TCM) and is associated with the Kidney organ and the urinary system. The Kidney meridian starts at the bottom of the foot and runs up the leg, through the torso and chest, and ends at the collarbone. Along its pathway, there are various acupoints that can be stimulated to promote the flow of Qi and restore balance to the body.

In TCM, the Kidneys are considered the organs responsible for the storage and circulation of Jing, which is believed to be the essence of life. The Kidney meridian is believed to regulate the flow of Qi in the body and maintain the balance between the interior and exterior environment. Stimulating the acupoints along the Kidney meridian can help promote the flow of Qi and restore balance to the body.

Kidney 3 is one of the key acupoints along the Kidney meridian and is located on the inner ankle. It is often used to treat fatigue and low back pain. Stimulating this acupoint is also believed to help strengthen the Kidneys and promote the flow of Qi and blood.

Another important acupoint along the Kidney meridian is Kidney 7, located on the foot, just above the inner ankle bone. This acupoint is often used to treat Kidney-related issues such as frequent urination and night sweats. Stimulating this acupoint is also believed to promote the flow of Qi and help reduce stress and tension in the body.

Kidney 27 is located on the chest, just below the collarbone, and is believed to be a key acupoint for the Kidney meridian. Stimulating this acupoint is often used to treat respiratory issues such as asthma and cough. It is also believed to promote the flow of Qi and help reduce stress and tension in the body.

In addition to acupuncture and acupressure, dietary therapy is also an essential aspect of TCM that can be used to support the Kidney meridian. Foods that are believed to support the Kidney meridian include black beans, kidney beans, and sesame seeds. These foods are believed to have a nourishing and strengthening effect on the body, which can help support the Kidneys and promote the flow of Qi and blood.

In TCM, the Kidney meridian is also associated with specific emotions, such as fear and anxiety. Imbalances in these emotions can lead to disruptions in the flow of Qi along the Kidney meridian and ultimately result in physical symptoms such as fatigue and low back pain.

TCM practitioners use various techniques, such as acupuncture and acupressure, to stimulate the flow of Qi along the Kidney meridian and restore balance to the body. Acupuncture involves the insertion of fine needles into specific acupoints along the meridian to promote the flow of Qi and restore balance. Acupressure is a similar technique that involves applying pressure to specific acupoints using the fingers, hands, or other tools.

The Pericardium Meridian

The Pericardium meridian is one of the twelve major meridians in Traditional Chinese Medicine (TCM) and is associated with the Pericardium organ and the cardiovascular system. The Pericardium meridian starts at the chest, near the nipple, and runs down the arm, through the wrist and hand, and ends at the tip of the middle finger. Along its pathway, there are various acupoints that can be stimulated to promote the flow of Qi and restore balance to the body.

In TCM, the Pericardium is considered the organ responsible for protecting the heart and regulating blood flow. The Pericardium meridian is believed to regulate the flow of Qi in the body and maintain the balance between the interior and exterior environment. Stimulating the acupoints along the Pericardium meridian can help promote the flow of Qi and restore balance to the body.

Pericardium 6 is one of the key acupoints along the Pericardium meridian and is located on the inner wrist, two finger-widths below the wrist crease. It is often used to treat nausea and vomiting, as well as anxiety and insomnia. Stimulating this acupoint is also believed to promote the flow of Qi and blood, and help reduce stress and tension in the body.

Another important acupoint along the Pericardium meridian is Pericardium 7, located on the wrist, in line with the little finger. This acupoint is often used to treat heart-related issues such as palpitations and chest pain. Stimulating this acupoint is also believed to promote the flow of Qi and help reduce stress and tension in the body.

Pericardium 8 is located on the palm of the hand, between the fourth and fifth fingers, and is believed to be a key acupoint for the Pericardium meridian. Stimulating this acupoint is often used to treat chest pain and promote relaxation. It is also believed to promote the flow of Qi and help reduce stress and tension in the body.

In addition to acupuncture and acupressure, dietary therapy is also an essential aspect of TCM that can be used to support the Pericardium meridian. Foods that are believed to support the Pericardium meridian include beets, cherries, and hawthorn berries. These foods are believed to have a nourishing and strengthening effect on the body, which can help support the cardiovascular system.

In TCM, the Pericardium meridian is also associated with specific emotions, such as joy and excitement. Imbalances in these emotions can lead to disruptions in the flow of Qi along the Pericardium meridian and ultimately result in physical symptoms such as chest pain and palpitations.

TCM practitioners use various techniques, such as acupuncture and acupressure, to stimulate the flow of Qi along the Pericardium meridian and restore balance to the body. Acupuncture involves the insertion of fine needles into specific acupoints along the meridian to promote the flow of Qi and restore balance. Acupressure is a similar technique that involves applying pressure to specific acupoints using the fingers, hands, or other tools.

The Triple Warmer Meridian

The Triple Warmer meridian is one of the twelve major meridians in Traditional Chinese Medicine (TCM) and is associated with the Triple Warmer organ and the body's defense systems. The Triple Warmer meridian starts at the ring finger and runs up the arm, through the shoulder, and ends at the temple. Along its pathway, there are various acupoints that can be stimulated to promote the flow of Qi and restore balance to the body.

In TCM, the Triple Warmer is considered the organ responsible for regulating the body's defense systems and coordinating the functions of the other organs. The Triple Warmer meridian is believed to regulate the flow of Qi in the body and maintain the balance between the interior and exterior environment. Stimulating the acupoints along the Triple Warmer meridian can help promote the flow of Qi and restore balance to the body.

Triple Warmer 5 is one of the key acupoints along the Triple Warmer meridian and is located on the outer wrist, just above the wrist joint. It is often used to treat wrist pain and stiffness, as well as shoulder pain and tension. Stimulating this acupoint is also believed to promote the flow of Qi and blood, and help reduce stress and tension in the body.

Another important acupoint along the Triple Warmer meridian is Triple Warmer 6, located on the outer forearm, three finger-widths above the wrist crease. This acupoint is often used to treat arm pain and tension, as well as headaches and dizziness. Stimulating this acupoint is also believed to promote the flow of Qi and help reduce stress and tension in the body.

Triple Warmer 23 is located at the temple and is believed to be a key acupoint for the Triple Warmer meridian. Stimulating this acupoint is often used to treat headaches, migraines, and eye pain. It is also believed to promote the flow of Qi and help reduce stress and tension in the body.

In addition to acupuncture and acupressure, dietary therapy is also an essential aspect of TCM that can be used to support the Triple Warmer meridian. Foods that are believed to support the Triple Warmer meridian include garlic, ginger, and green tea. These foods are believed to have a warming and stimulating effect on the body, which can help support the immune system and promote overall well-being.

In TCM, the Triple Warmer meridian is also associated with specific emotions, such as fear and anxiety. Imbalances in these emotions can lead to disruptions in the flow of Qi along the Triple Warmer meridian and ultimately result in physical symptoms such as pain and tension in the body.

TCM practitioners use various techniques, such as acupuncture and acupressure, to stimulate the flow of Qi along the Triple Warmer meridian and restore balance to the body. Acupuncture involves the insertion of fine needles into specific acupoints along the meridian to promote the flow of Qi and restore balance. Acupressure is a similar technique that involves applying pressure to specific acupoints using the fingers, hands, or other tools.

The Gallbladder Meridian

The Gallbladder meridian is one of the twelve major meridians in Traditional Chinese Medicine (TCM) and is associated with the Gallbladder organ and the digestive system. The Gallbladder meridian starts at the outer corner of the eye and runs down the side of the head and neck, through the shoulder and hip, and ends at the fourth toe. Along its pathway, there are various acupoints that can be stimulated to promote the flow of Qi and restore balance to the body.

In TCM, the Gallbladder is considered the organ responsible for storing and secreting bile to aid in digestion. The Gallbladder meridian is believed to regulate the flow of Qi in the body and maintain the balance between the interior and exterior environment. Stimulating the acupoints along the Gallbladder meridian can help promote the flow of Qi and restore balance to the body.

Gallbladder 20 is one of the key acupoints along the Gallbladder meridian and is located at the base of the skull, in the hollows on either side of the spine. It is often used to treat headaches, neck pain, and tension. Stimulating this acupoint is also believed to promote the flow of Qi and blood, and help reduce stress and tension in the body.

Another important acupoint along the Gallbladder meridian is Gallbladder 30, located on the buttocks, just below the hip bone. This acupoint is often used to treat hip pain and stiffness, as well as sciatica. Stimulating this acupoint is also believed to promote the flow of Qi and help reduce stress and tension in the body.

Gallbladder 34 is located on the outer leg, just below the knee, and is believed to be a key acupoint for the Gallbladder meridian. Stimulating this acupoint is often used to treat knee pain, as well as digestive issues such as nausea and vomiting. It is also believed to promote the flow of Qi and help reduce stress and tension in the body.

In addition to acupuncture and acupressure, dietary therapy is also an essential aspect of TCM that can be used to support the Gallbladder meridian. Foods that are believed to support the Gallbladder meridian include beets, carrots, and dandelion greens. These foods are believed to have a cleansing and detoxifying effect on the body, which can help support the digestive system.

In TCM, the Gallbladder meridian is also associated with specific emotions, such as decision-making and courage. Imbalances in these emotions can lead to disruptions in the flow of Qi along the Gallbladder meridian and ultimately result in physical symptoms such as pain and tension in the body.

TCM practitioners use various techniques, such as acupuncture and acupressure, to stimulate the flow of Qi along the Gallbladder meridian and restore balance to the body. Acupuncture involves the insertion of fine needles into specific acupoints along the meridian to promote the flow of Qi and restore balance. Acupressure is a similar technique that involves applying pressure to specific acupoints using the fingers, hands, or other tools.

The Liver Meridian

The Liver meridian is one of the twelve major meridians in Traditional Chinese Medicine (TCM) and is associated with the Liver organ and the body's detoxification system. The Liver meridian starts at the big toe and runs up the inside of the leg, through the abdomen, and ends at the fourth rib. Along its pathway, there are various acupoints that can be stimulated to promote the flow of Qi and restore balance to the body.

In TCM, the Liver is considered the organ responsible for regulating the flow of Qi in the body and storing blood. The Liver meridian is believed to regulate the flow of Qi in the body and maintain the balance between the interior and exterior environment. Stimulating the acupoints along the Liver meridian can help promote the flow of Qi and restore balance to the body.

Liver 3 is one of the key acupoints along the Liver meridian and is located on the foot, between the big toe and second toe. It is often used to treat headaches, menstrual cramps, and digestive issues. Stimulating this acupoint is also believed to promote the flow of Qi and blood, and help reduce stress and tension in the body.

Another important acupoint along the Liver meridian is Liver 13, located on the abdomen, just below the ribcage. This acupoint is often used to treat digestive issues such as bloating and indigestion, as well as menstrual cramps. Stimulating this acupoint is also believed to promote the flow of Qi and help reduce stress and tension in the body.

Liver 14 is located on the chest, just below the nipple and is believed to be a key acupoint for the Liver meridian. Stimulating this acupoint is often used to treat chest pain and tension, as well as menstrual cramps. It is also believed to promote the flow of Qi and help reduce stress and tension in the body.

In addition to acupuncture and acupressure, dietary therapy is also an essential aspect of TCM that can be used to support the Liver meridian. Foods that are believed to support the Liver meridian include dark leafy greens, citrus fruits, and ginger. These foods are believed to have a cleansing and detoxifying effect on the body, which can help support the liver and promote overall well-being.

In TCM, the Liver meridian is also associated with specific emotions, such as anger and frustration. Imbalances in these emotions can lead to disruptions in the flow of Qi along the Liver meridian and ultimately result in physical symptoms such as pain and tension in the body.

TCM practitioners use various techniques, such as acupuncture and acupressure, to stimulate the flow of Qi along the Liver meridian and restore balance to the body. Acupuncture involves the insertion of fine needles into specific acupoints along the meridian to promote the flow of Qi and restore balance. Acupressure is a similar technique that involves applying pressure to specific acupoints using the fingers, hands, or other tools.

Yin and Yang Meridians

In Traditional Chinese Medicine (TCM), the concept of Yin and Yang is fundamental to understanding the body's energy balance. Yin represents the feminine, receptive, and nourishing aspect of energy, while Yang represents the masculine, active, and stimulating aspect of energy. The twelve major meridians in TCM are divided into six Yin meridians and six Yang meridians, each with its own unique properties and functions.

The Yin meridians are associated with the internal organs and are responsible for nourishing and replenishing the body. The six Yin meridians are the Lung, Spleen, Heart, Kidney, Pericardium, and Liver meridians.

The Lung meridian, for example, is associated with the lungs and is responsible for regulating the flow of Qi and breathing. The Spleen meridian is associated with the digestive system and is responsible for transforming food into Qi and blood. The Heart meridian is associated with the heart and is responsible for regulating the circulation of blood and emotions. The Kidney meridian is associated with the kidneys and is responsible for regulating the body's water metabolism and reproductive functions. The Pericardium meridian is associated with the heart protector and is responsible for regulating the emotions and the flow of Qi in the chest. The Liver meridian is associated with the liver and is responsible for regulating the flow of Qi and blood and detoxifying the body.

On the other hand, the Yang meridians are associated with the external and functional aspects of the body and are responsible for providing energy and protection. The six Yang meridians are the Large Intestine, Stomach, Small Intestine, Bladder, Triple Warmer, and Gallbladder meridians.

The Large Intestine meridian is associated with the colon and is responsible for regulating the elimination of waste from the body. The Stomach meridian is associated with the stomach and is responsible for transforming food into Qi and blood. The Small Intestine meridian is associated with the small intestine and is responsible for separating the pure from the impure in the digestion process. The Bladder meridian is associated with the bladder and is responsible for regulating the flow of urine and water metabolism. The Triple Warmer meridian is associated with the body's three warmer regions and is responsible for regulating the body's temperature and energy. The Gallbladder meridian is associated with the gallbladder and is responsible for storing and secreting bile to aid in digestion.

Stimulating the Yin and Yang meridians through acupuncture and acupressure can help to balance the body's energy and promote overall well-being. For example, if a person is experiencing symptoms of excess heat, such as inflammation or fever, the acupoints along the Yin meridians can be stimulated to help cool the body and reduce inflammation. If a person is experiencing symptoms of weakness or fatigue, the acupoints along the Yang meridians can be stimulated to help boost energy and vitality.

In addition to acupuncture and acupressure, other TCM practices such as herbal medicine, dietary therapy, and qigong can also be used to balance the Yin and Yang meridians and promote overall health and wellness.

The Concept of Yin and Yang

The concept of Yin and Yang is a fundamental principle in Traditional Chinese Medicine (TCM) that is used to understand the balance and harmony of the body's energy. Yin and Yang are two opposing yet complementary forces that exist in all aspects of life, including the human body.

In TCM, the twelve major meridians are divided into six Yin meridians and six Yang meridians. The Yin meridians are associated with the internal organs and are responsible for nourishing and replenishing the body. The Yang meridians are associated with the external and functional aspects of the body and are responsible for providing energy and protection.

The Yin meridians are associated with the feminine, receptive, and nourishing aspects of energy. Yin represents the darker, colder, and more passive qualities in the body. The Yin meridians are responsible for nourishing and replenishing the body's energy and fluids, regulating the emotions, and supporting the internal organs.

The six Yin meridians are the Lung, Spleen, Heart, Kidney, Pericardium, and Liver meridians. The Lung meridian is responsible for regulating the flow of Qi and breathing. The Spleen meridian is responsible for transforming food into Qi and blood. The Heart meridian is responsible for regulating the circulation of blood and emotions. The Kidney meridian is responsible for regulating the body's water metabolism and reproductive functions. The Pericardium meridian is responsible for regulating the emotions and the flow of Qi in the chest. The Liver meridian is responsible for regulating the flow of Qi and blood and detoxifying the body.

The Yang meridians are associated with the masculine, active, and stimulating aspects of energy. Yang represents the brighter, warmer, and more active qualities in the body. The Yang meridians are responsible for providing energy and protection to the body, regulating the body's temperature, and promoting circulation.

The six Yang meridians are the Large Intestine, Stomach, Small Intestine, Bladder, Triple Warmer, and Gallbladder meridians. The Large Intestine meridian is responsible for regulating the elimination of waste from the body. The Stomach meridian is responsible for transforming food into Qi and blood. The Small Intestine meridian is responsible for separating the pure from the impure in the digestion process. The Bladder meridian is responsible for regulating the flow of urine and water metabolism. The Triple Warmer meridian is responsible for regulating the body's temperature and energy. The Gallbladder meridian is responsible for storing and secreting bile to aid in digestion.

In TCM, the balance between Yin and Yang is essential to maintain the body's health and wellness. An imbalance in Yin and Yang can lead to physical and emotional disorders. TCM practitioners use various techniques, such as acupuncture and herbal medicine, to restore the balance between Yin and Yang and promote overall well-being.

Acupuncture is a technique that involves the insertion of fine needles into specific acupoints along the meridians to promote the flow of Qi and restore balance. The selection of acupoints depends on the individual's specific symptoms and imbalances. For example, if a person is experiencing symptoms of excess heat, such as inflammation or fever, the acupoints along the Yin meridians can be stimulated to help cool the body and reduce inflammation. If a person is experiencing symptoms of weakness or fatigue, the acupoints along the Yang meridians can be stimulated to help boost energy and vitality.

Herbal medicine is another technique used in TCM to balance Yin and Yang. Certain herbs are believed to have Yin or Yang properties and can be prescribed to restore the balance between the two forces.

The Relationship Between Yin and Yang Meridians

In Traditional Chinese Medicine (TCM), the concept of Yin and Yang is essential to understanding the body's energy balance. Yin and Yang are two opposing yet complementary forces that exist in all aspects of life, including the human body. The twelve major meridians in TCM are divided into six Yin meridians and six Yang meridians, each with its own unique properties and functions.

The Yin meridians are associated with the internal organs and are responsible for nourishing and replenishing the body. The six Yin meridians are the Lung, Spleen, Heart, Kidney, Pericardium, and Liver meridians. The Yang meridians are associated with the external and functional aspects of the body and are responsible for providing energy and protection. The six Yang meridians are the Large Intestine, Stomach, Small Intestine, Bladder, Triple Warmer, and Gallbladder meridians.

The Yin and Yang meridians are interconnected and work together to maintain the body's balance and harmony. When one meridian is imbalanced, it can affect the corresponding meridian and disrupt the balance between Yin and Yang.

For example, the Lung meridian, which is a Yin meridian, is responsible for regulating the flow of Qi and breathing. If the Lung meridian is imbalanced, it can affect the corresponding Yang meridian, the Large Intestine meridian, which is responsible for regulating the elimination of waste from the body. An imbalance in the Lung meridian can lead to symptoms such as coughing, wheezing, and shortness of breath, which can then affect the Large Intestine meridian, causing symptoms such as constipation or diarrhea.

Similarly, the Liver meridian, which is a Yin meridian, is responsible for regulating the flow of Qi and blood and detoxifying the body. If the Liver meridian is imbalanced, it can affect the corresponding Yang meridian, the Gallbladder meridian, which is responsible for storing and secreting bile to aid in digestion. An imbalance in the Liver meridian can lead to symptoms such as headaches, irritability, and mood swings, which can then affect the Gallbladder meridian, causing symptoms such as nausea or indigestion.

To restore balance between the Yin and Yang meridians, TCM practitioners use various techniques, such as acupuncture and herbal medicine. Acupuncture involves the insertion of fine needles into specific acupoints along the meridians to promote the flow of Qi and restore balance. The selection of acupoints depends on the individual's specific symptoms and imbalances. Herbal medicine is another technique used in TCM to balance Yin and Yang. Certain herbs are believed to have Yin or Yang properties and can be prescribed to restore the balance between the two forces.

In addition to acupuncture and herbal medicine, other TCM practices such as dietary therapy and qigong can also be used to balance the Yin and Yang meridians and promote overall health and wellness. Dietary therapy involves the use of food as medicine to balance the body's energy and nourish the organs. Qigong is a form of gentle exercise that involves breathing techniques, meditation, and movements to promote the flow of Qi and balance the body's energy.

The Five Elements and Meridians

The Five Elements Theory is an important concept in Traditional Chinese Medicine (TCM) that is used to understand the relationship between the human body and the natural world. The theory describes five basic elements, which are wood, fire, earth, metal, and water, that represent different aspects of nature and the human body. Each element is associated with specific meridians and organs in the body, and the balance between the elements is essential for maintaining health and preventing disease.

In TCM, the twelve major meridians are divided into six Yin meridians and six Yang meridians. Each meridian is associated with specific organs and functions in the body. The meridians are also associated with the Five Elements Theory, which helps to explain their functions and relationships.

The Wood Element is associated with the Liver and Gallbladder meridians. The Liver meridian is responsible for regulating the flow of Qi and blood, detoxifying the body, and storing and releasing blood. The Gallbladder meridian is responsible for storing and secreting bile to aid in digestion. The Wood Element is also associated with the energy of growth, expansion, and creativity.

The Fire Element is associated with the Heart and Small Intestine meridians. The Heart meridian is responsible for regulating the circulation of blood and emotions, while the Small Intestine meridian is responsible for separating the pure from the impure in the digestion process. The Fire Element is also associated with the energy of warmth, passion, and connection.

The Earth Element is associated with the Spleen and Stomach meridians. The Spleen meridian is responsible for transforming food into Qi and blood, while the Stomach meridian is responsible for breaking down food and transporting it to the Small Intestine. The Earth Element is also associated with the energy of nurturing, stability, and groundedness.

The Metal Element is associated with the Lung and Large Intestine meridians. The Lung meridian is responsible for regulating the flow of Qi and breathing, while the Large Intestine meridian is responsible for regulating the elimination of waste from the body. The Metal Element is also associated with the energy of clarity, precision, and order.

The Water Element is associated with the Kidney and Bladder meridians. The Kidney meridian is responsible for regulating the body's water metabolism and reproductive functions, while the Bladder meridian is responsible for regulating the flow of urine and water metabolism. The Water Element is also associated with the energy of deep wisdom, fluidity, and adaptability.

The Five Elements Theory provides a framework for understanding the relationships between the meridians and organs in the body. The theory helps to explain how imbalances in one element can affect the corresponding meridians and organs, as well as other aspects of the body and mind.

For example, an imbalance in the Wood Element, which is associated with the Liver and Gallbladder meridians, can lead to symptoms such as anger, frustration, and digestive problems. Similarly, an imbalance in the Water Element, which is associated with the Kidney and Bladder meridians, can lead to symptoms such as fear, fatigue, and reproductive issues.

To restore balance between the elements and meridians, TCM practitioners use various techniques, such as acupuncture, herbal medicine, and dietary therapy. Acupuncture involves the insertion of fine needles into specific acupoints along the meridians to promote the flow of Qi and restore balance. Herbal medicine is another technique used in TCM to balance the elements and meridians. Certain herbs are believed to have specific properties that can be used to balance the different elements and restore harmony in the body.

Introduction to the Five Elements

The Five Elements Theory is a fundamental concept in Traditional Chinese Medicine (TCM) that is used to explain the relationship between the human body and the natural world. The theory describes five basic elements, which are wood, fire, earth, metal, and water, that represent different aspects of nature and the human body. Each element is associated with specific meridians and organs in the body, and the balance between the elements is essential for maintaining health and preventing disease.

In TCM, the human body is seen as a microcosm of the natural world, and the Five Elements Theory is used to explain the interconnections between different aspects of the body and mind. The theory is based on the observation that each of the five elements has a specific set of characteristics that can be used to describe different aspects of the human experience.

The Wood Element is associated with the energy of growth, expansion, and creativity. It is associated with the Liver and Gallbladder meridians, which are responsible for regulating the flow of Qi and blood, detoxifying the body, and aiding in digestion.

The Fire Element is associated with the energy of warmth, passion, and connection. It is associated with the Heart and Small Intestine meridians, which are responsible for regulating the circulation of blood and emotions, and separating the pure from the impure in the digestion process.

The Earth Element is associated with the energy of nurturing, stability, and groundedness. It is associated with the Spleen and Stomach meridians, which are responsible for transforming food into Qi and blood, breaking down food, and transporting it to the Small Intestine.

The Metal Element is associated with the energy of clarity, precision, and order. It is associated with the Lung and Large Intestine meridians, which are responsible for regulating the flow of Qi and breathing, and regulating the elimination of waste from the body.

The Water Element is associated with the energy of deep wisdom, fluidity, and adaptability. It is associated with the Kidney and Bladder meridians, which are responsible for regulating the body's water metabolism, reproductive functions, and urinary system.

The Five Elements Theory provides a framework for understanding the relationships between different aspects of the body and mind. For example, an imbalance in the Wood Element can lead to symptoms such as anger, frustration, and digestive problems, while an imbalance in the Water Element can lead to symptoms such as fear, fatigue, and reproductive issues.

To restore balance between the elements, TCM practitioners use various techniques, such as acupuncture, herbal medicine, and dietary therapy. Acupuncture involves the insertion of fine needles into specific acupoints along the meridians to promote the flow of Qi and restore balance. Herbal medicine is another technique used in TCM to balance the elements. Certain herbs are believed to have specific properties that can be used to balance the different elements and restore harmony in the body.

Dietary therapy is another important aspect of TCM that is used to balance the elements. Different foods are believed to have specific properties that can be used to balance the different elements and promote overall health and wellness. For example, foods that are associated with the Earth Element, such as grains, vegetables, and legumes, are believed to be nourishing and grounding, while foods that are associated with the Fire Element, such as spicy foods, are believed to be warming and invigorating.

The Relationship Between Meridians and the Five Elements

The Five Elements Theory is an important concept in Traditional Chinese Medicine (TCM) that helps to explain the relationship between the human body and the natural world. The theory describes five basic elements, which are wood, fire, earth, metal, and water, that represent different aspects of nature and the human body. Each element is associated with specific meridians and organs in the body, and the balance between the elements is essential for maintaining health and preventing disease.

In TCM, the twelve major meridians are divided into six Yin meridians and six Yang meridians. Each meridian is associated with specific organs and functions in the body. The meridians are also associated with the Five Elements Theory, which helps to explain their functions and relationships.

The Wood Element is associated with the Liver and Gallbladder meridians. The Liver meridian is responsible for regulating the flow of Qi and blood, detoxifying the body, and storing and releasing blood. The Gallbladder meridian is responsible for storing and secreting bile to aid in digestion. The Wood Element is also associated with the energy of growth, expansion, and creativity.

The Fire Element is associated with the Heart and Small Intestine meridians. The Heart meridian is responsible for regulating the circulation of blood and emotions, while the Small Intestine meridian is responsible for separating the pure from the impure in the digestion process. The Fire Element is also associated with the energy of warmth, passion, and connection.

The Earth Element is associated with the Spleen and Stomach meridians. The Spleen meridian is responsible for transforming food into Qi and blood, while the Stomach meridian is responsible for breaking down food and transporting it to the Small Intestine. The Earth Element is also associated with the energy of nurturing, stability, and groundedness.

The Metal Element is associated with the Lung and Large Intestine meridians. The Lung meridian is responsible for regulating the flow of Qi and breathing, while the Large Intestine meridian is responsible for regulating the elimination of waste from the body. The Metal Element is also associated with the energy of clarity, precision, and order.

The Water Element is associated with the Kidney and Bladder meridians. The Kidney meridian is responsible for regulating the body's water metabolism and reproductive functions, while the Bladder meridian is responsible for regulating the flow of urine and water metabolism. The Water Element is also associated with the energy of deep wisdom, fluidity, and adaptability.

The Five Elements Theory provides a framework for understanding the relationships between the meridians and organs in the body. The theory helps to explain how imbalances in one element can affect the corresponding meridians and organs, as well as other aspects of the body and mind.

For example, an imbalance in the Wood Element, which is associated with the Liver and Gallbladder meridians, can lead to symptoms such as anger, frustration, and digestive problems. Similarly, an imbalance in the Water Element, which is associated with the Kidney and Bladder meridians, can lead to symptoms such as fear, fatigue, and reproductive issues.

To restore balance between the elements and meridians, TCM practitioners use various techniques, such as acupuncture, herbal medicine, and dietary therapy. Acupuncture involves the insertion of fine needles into specific acupoints along the meridians to promote the flow of Qi and restore balance. Herbal medicine is another technique used in TCM to balance the elements and meridians. Certain herbs are believed to have specific properties that can be used to balance the different elements and restore harmony in the body.

The Meridian Clock

The Meridian Clock, also known as the Body Clock or Organ Clock, is a concept in Traditional Chinese Medicine (TCM) that describes the relationship between the twelve major meridians and the organs they are associated with. The Meridian Clock is based on the idea that each meridian has a two-hour period of peak activity during a 24-hour day, and that imbalances in the meridians can lead to health problems.

The Meridian Clock is divided into twelve two-hour periods, with each period representing one of the twelve meridians. The Meridian Clock begins at 3am with the Lung meridian, followed by the Large Intestine, Stomach, Spleen, Heart, Small Intestine, Bladder, Kidney, Pericardium, Triple Warmer, Gallbladder, and Liver meridians. Each meridian has a two-hour period of maximum activity, followed by a two-hour period of minimum activity.

The Lung meridian is active from 3am to 5am, and is associated with the respiratory system and the immune system. The Large Intestine meridian is active from 5am to 7am, and is associated with the elimination of waste from the body. The Stomach meridian is active from 7am to 9am, and is associated with digestion and the processing of nutrients.

The Spleen meridian is active from 9am to 11am, and is associated with the production of Qi and blood, as well as the distribution of nutrients to the body. The Heart meridian is active from 11am to 1pm, and is associated with circulation and emotional well-being. The Small Intestine meridian is active from 1pm to 3pm, and is associated with the separation of the pure from the impure in the digestion process.

The Bladder meridian is active from 3pm to 5pm, and is associated with the elimination of waste and the regulation of the body's water metabolism. The Kidney meridian is active from 5pm to 7pm, and is associated with the body's water metabolism and reproductive functions. The Pericardium meridian is active from 7pm to 9pm, and is associated with the heart and emotional well-being.

The Triple Warmer meridian is active from 9pm to 11pm, and is associated with the body's energy metabolism and the regulation of body temperature. The Gallbladder meridian is active from 11pm to 1am, and is associated with the digestion of fats and the storage and secretion of bile. The Liver meridian is active from 1am to 3am, and is associated with the regulation of the body's Qi and blood.

The Meridian Clock is an important concept in TCM that helps to explain the relationship between the body's internal organs and the external environment. According to TCM, the body is influenced by external factors such as weather, seasons, and time of day, and these factors can affect the body's internal balance.

Imbalances in the meridians can lead to a variety of health problems, such as pain, fatigue, digestive problems, and emotional issues. TCM practitioners use various techniques, such as acupuncture, herbal medicine, and dietary therapy, to balance the meridians and restore health.

Acupuncture involves the insertion of fine needles into specific acupoints along the meridians to promote the flow of Qi and restore balance. Herbal medicine is another technique used in TCM to balance the meridians. Certain herbs are believed to have specific properties that can be used to balance the different meridians and restore harmony in the body.

The Concept of the Meridian Clock

The Meridian Clock, also known as the Body Clock or Organ Clock, is a concept in Traditional Chinese Medicine (TCM) that describes the relationship between the twelve major meridians and the organs they are associated with. The Meridian Clock is based on the idea that each meridian has a two-hour period of peak activity during a 24-hour day, and that imbalances in the meridians can lead to health problems.

The concept of the Meridian Clock is a fundamental aspect of TCM and has been used for centuries to diagnose and treat a variety of health conditions. According to TCM, the body is influenced by external factors such as weather, seasons, and time of day, and these factors can affect the body's internal balance.

The Meridian Clock is divided into twelve two-hour periods, with each period representing one of the twelve meridians. The Meridian Clock begins at 3am with the Lung meridian, followed by the Large Intestine, Stomach, Spleen, Heart, Small Intestine, Bladder, Kidney, Pericardium, Triple Warmer, Gallbladder, and Liver meridians. Each meridian has a two-hour period of maximum activity, followed by a two-hour period of minimum activity.

The Meridian Clock is an important diagnostic tool in TCM, and practitioners use it to identify imbalances in the meridians and organs. For example, if a patient complains of frequent waking between 3am and 5am, this may indicate an imbalance in the Lung meridian. If a patient has digestive problems between 7am and 9am, this may indicate an imbalance in the Stomach meridian.

TCM practitioners use various techniques to balance the meridians and restore health. Acupuncture involves the insertion of fine needles into specific acupoints along the meridians to promote the flow of Qi and restore balance. Herbal medicine is another technique used in TCM to balance the meridians. Certain herbs are believed to have specific properties that can be used to balance the different meridians and restore harmony in the body.

Dietary therapy is another important aspect of TCM. According to TCM, different foods have different properties and can be used to balance the meridians and promote health. For example, if a patient has an imbalance in the Spleen meridian, they may be advised to eat foods that are warm and nourishing, such as soups and stews.

The Meridian Clock is also used in TCM to guide the timing of certain activities, such as exercise and meditation. For example, if a patient wants to improve their respiratory health, they may be advised to practice breathing exercises during the two-hour period when the Lung meridian is most active. Similarly, if a patient wants to improve their emotional well-being, they may be advised to practice meditation during the two-hour period when the Heart meridian is most active.

In addition to the daily Meridian Clock, there is also a yearly Meridian Clock that corresponds to the seasons. According to TCM, each season is associated with a specific organ and meridian. For example, the Liver meridian is associated with the spring season, while the Lung meridian is associated with the fall season. TCM practitioners use the yearly Meridian Clock to guide treatments and lifestyle recommendations throughout the year.

The concept of the Meridian Clock is a unique aspect of TCM that has been used for centuries to diagnose and treat a variety of health conditions. While there is still much research to be done on the science behind the Meridian Clock, many people have reported significant improvements in their health and well-being after receiving TCM treatments that take the Meridian Clock into account.

How to Use the Meridian Clock for Optimal Health

The Meridian Clock, also known as the Body Clock or Organ Clock, is a concept in Traditional Chinese Medicine (TCM) that describes the relationship between the twelve major meridians and the organs they are associated with. By understanding the Meridian Clock and how it relates to the body's internal balance, you can use this knowledge to optimize your health and well-being.

To use the Meridian Clock for optimal health, it's important to first understand the twelve major meridians and their associated organs. The meridians are the pathways through which Qi, or vital energy, flows through the body. Each meridian is associated with a specific organ and has a two-hour period of peak activity during a 24-hour day. The Meridian Clock begins at 3am with the Lung meridian, followed by the Large Intestine, Stomach, Spleen, Heart, Small Intestine, Bladder, Kidney, Pericardium, Triple Warmer, Gallbladder, and Liver meridians.

Here are some tips on how to use the Meridian Clock for optimal health:

Sleep and Wake Up at the Right Time

According to the Meridian Clock, the best time to wake up is between 5am and 7am, during the two-hour period when the Large Intestine meridian is most active. This is because the Large Intestine meridian is associated with elimination and detoxification, and waking up during this time can help promote bowel movements and remove waste from the body.

The best time to go to bed is between 9pm and 11pm, during the two-hour period when the Gallbladder meridian is most active. The Gallbladder meridian is associated with decision-making and judgment, and going to bed during this time can help you make better decisions and sleep more soundly.

Eat at the Right Time

Eating at the right time can help promote digestion and absorption of nutrients. According to the Meridian Clock, the best time to have breakfast is between 7am and 9am, during the two-hour period when the Stomach meridian is most active. The Stomach meridian is associated with digestion and nourishment, and having breakfast during this time can help promote healthy digestion and provide energy for the day.

The best time to have lunch is between 11am and 1pm, during the two-hour period when the Heart meridian is most active. The Heart meridian is associated with circulation and nourishment, and having lunch during this time can help promote healthy blood flow and provide nutrients to the body.

The best time to have dinner is between 5pm and 7pm, during the two-hour period when the Pericardium meridian is most active. The Pericardium meridian is associated with digestion and absorption, and having dinner during this time can help promote healthy digestion and ensure that nutrients are properly absorbed.

Exercise at the Right Time

Exercising at the right time can help promote physical and mental health. According to the Meridian Clock, the best time to exercise is between 7am and 9am, during the two-hour period when the Stomach meridian is most active. The Stomach meridian is associated with digestion and nourishment, and exercising during this time can help promote healthy digestion and provide energy for the day.

If you prefer to exercise in the evening, the best time to do so is between 5pm and 7pm, during the two-hour period when the Pericardium meridian is most active. The Pericardium meridian is associated with circulation and nourishment, and exercising during this time can help promote healthy blood flow and provide nutrients to the body.

Meridian Diagnosis and Assessment

Meridian diagnosis and assessment is an essential component of Traditional Chinese Medicine (TCM) and involves the evaluation of the body's energy flow through the twelve major meridians. The meridians are pathways through which vital energy or Qi flows throughout the body, and blockages or imbalances in these meridians can lead to various health issues. Meridian diagnosis and assessment can help TCM practitioners identify these blockages and imbalances and develop treatment plans to restore the body's natural balance.

The twelve major meridians are associated with specific organs and have corresponding acupressure points that can be evaluated during meridian diagnosis and assessment. These acupressure points are located along the meridian pathways and can be palpated to evaluate the energy flow in the meridian.

During a meridian diagnosis and assessment, a TCM practitioner will examine each of the twelve major meridians and their associated organs to identify any blockages or imbalances. They may also evaluate other factors such as the patient's pulse, tongue, and overall physical and emotional state to develop a complete understanding of the patient's condition.

Here are some of the main techniques used in meridian diagnosis and assessment:

Pulse Diagnosis

Pulse diagnosis is a technique used in TCM to evaluate the energy flow in the body. During a pulse diagnosis, the practitioner will take the patient's pulse at three different locations on each wrist, evaluating the strength and quality of the pulse at each location. This can provide information about the energy flow in the twelve major meridians and the corresponding organs.

Tongue Diagnosis

Tongue diagnosis is another technique used in TCM to evaluate the body's energy flow. The practitioner will examine the patient's tongue, evaluating its color, shape, coating, and moisture. This can provide information about the state of the body's organs and meridians.

Palpation of Acupressure Points

During a meridian diagnosis and assessment, the practitioner will palpate specific acupressure points along the meridian pathways to evaluate the energy flow in the meridian. They will apply pressure to these points and evaluate the patient's response to determine if there are any blockages or imbalances.

Observation of Physical and Emotional Symptoms

The practitioner may also observe the patient's physical and emotional symptoms to evaluate the energy flow in the body. For example, a patient with insomnia may indicate an imbalance in the Heart meridian, while a patient with digestive issues may indicate an imbalance in the Stomach or Large Intestine meridians.

Once the TCM practitioner has completed the meridian diagnosis and assessment, they will develop a treatment plan to address any blockages or imbalances identified. This may include acupuncture, acupressure, herbal remedies, dietary changes, and lifestyle modifications.

The Importance of Meridian Diagnosis

Meridian diagnosis is a key component of Traditional Chinese Medicine (TCM), which views the body as a network of energy channels or meridians. These meridians allow the flow of vital energy or Qi throughout the body, and imbalances or blockages in these pathways can lead to various health issues. Meridian diagnosis is used to assess the flow of energy through the body's meridians and identify any imbalances or blockages.

The human body has twelve major meridians, each associated with a specific organ system. These meridians are interconnected and work together to maintain the body's balance and overall health. When there is a disruption in the flow of energy through these meridians, it can lead to a range of physical and emotional symptoms.

Meridian diagnosis involves a thorough assessment of the body's energy flow through these meridians to determine where imbalances or blockages may be occurring. Practitioners of TCM use various techniques to evaluate the flow of energy, including pulse diagnosis, tongue diagnosis, and palpation of acupressure points.

Pulse diagnosis involves taking the patient's pulse at three different locations on each wrist and evaluating the strength and quality of the pulse at each location. The pulse provides information about the energy flow in the body's meridians and corresponding organs. A weak or irregular pulse may indicate an imbalance or blockage in the corresponding meridian.

Tongue diagnosis involves examining the patient's tongue to evaluate its color, shape, coating, and moisture. The tongue provides information about the state of the body's organs and meridians. A thick, yellow coating may indicate an imbalance in the Stomach or Large Intestine meridians, while a red tongue with a cracked surface may indicate an imbalance in the Heart meridian.

Palpation of acupressure points involves applying pressure to specific points along the meridian pathways to evaluate the energy flow in the meridian. The practitioner will palpate these points and evaluate the patient's response to determine if there are any blockages or imbalances.

By using these techniques, TCM practitioners can identify imbalances or blockages in the body's meridians and develop a treatment plan to restore the body's natural balance. Treatment may involve acupuncture, acupressure, herbal remedies, dietary changes, and lifestyle modifications.

Meridian diagnosis can be particularly useful in identifying imbalances or blockages that may not be apparent through other diagnostic methods. For example, a patient with chronic fatigue may have normal blood tests and physical exams, but a meridian diagnosis may reveal an imbalance in the Kidney or Spleen meridians, which are associated with energy production and metabolism.

Meridian diagnosis can also help TCM practitioners understand the underlying causes of a patient's symptoms, rather than just treating the symptoms themselves. By addressing the root cause of a patient's imbalance, TCM can promote long-term healing and prevent the recurrence of symptoms.

Methods for Assessing Meridian Health

Traditional Chinese Medicine (TCM) uses various methods for assessing meridian health to determine the flow of Qi or energy in the body's meridians. These methods include pulse diagnosis, tongue diagnosis, and palpation of acupressure points. Each of these methods provides valuable information about the state of the body's meridians and organs and helps TCM practitioners develop an effective treatment plan.

Pulse Diagnosis

Pulse diagnosis is a key method for assessing meridian health in TCM. The practitioner will take the patient's pulse at three locations on each wrist and evaluate the strength, quality, and rhythm of the pulse. Each location corresponds to a specific meridian and organ system, allowing the practitioner to assess the flow of energy through these channels.

The pulse is assessed on three levels: superficial, middle, and deep. The superficial pulse provides information about the Qi flow in the body's exterior, while the middle pulse reflects the state of the internal organs. The deep pulse provides information about the state of the bone marrow and reproductive organs.

Pulse diagnosis can reveal imbalances in the body's meridians and organs, such as a weak or irregular pulse indicating a blockage or deficiency in the corresponding meridian.

Tongue Diagnosis

Tongue diagnosis is another method for assessing meridian health in TCM. The practitioner will examine the patient's tongue to evaluate its color, shape, coating, and moisture. Each of these factors provides valuable information about the state of the body's meridians and organs.

The tongue's color can reveal imbalances in the body's meridians and organs. For example, a pale tongue may indicate a deficiency in Qi or blood, while a red tongue may indicate excess heat in the body.

The tongue's shape can also provide valuable information about meridian health. A swollen tongue may indicate an accumulation of dampness in the body, while a thin or pointed tongue may indicate a deficiency of Qi or blood.

The tongue's coating can reveal imbalances in the body's meridians and organs. For example, a thick, yellow coating may indicate an imbalance in the Stomach or Large Intestine meridians, while a white coating may indicate an imbalance in the Lung or Spleen meridians.

Palpation of Acupressure Points

Palpation of acupressure points is another method for assessing meridian health in TCM. The practitioner will apply pressure to specific points along the meridian pathways and evaluate the patient's response. The patient's response can reveal imbalances in the body's meridians and organs.

For example, a tender or sensitive point may indicate an imbalance or blockage in the corresponding meridian. The practitioner may also evaluate the patient's response to pressure on other acupressure points to assess the overall flow of energy in the body's meridians.

Other Methods for Assessing Meridian Health

In addition to pulse diagnosis, tongue diagnosis, and palpation of acupressure points, TCM also uses other methods for assessing meridian health. These include observation of the patient's physical appearance, such as the color and texture of their skin, and listening to the patient's voice to evaluate the state of the lungs and throat.

TCM practitioners may also ask the patient about their lifestyle habits, such as their diet, exercise routine, and sleep patterns, to gain a better understanding of the underlying causes of any imbalances in the body's meridians.

Acupressure Techniques

Acupressure is a form of traditional Chinese medicine (TCM) that involves applying pressure to specific points on the body to promote healing and balance in the body's energy flow, also known as Qi. Acupressure techniques can be used to treat a wide range of conditions, including pain, stress, anxiety, and digestive disorders. The techniques are based on the same principles as acupuncture, but instead of using needles, pressure is applied using the fingers, hands, or other devices.

Acupressure points are located along the body's meridians, which are the channels through which Qi flows. The meridians correspond to specific organs and systems in the body, and by applying pressure to the appropriate points, acupressure can help restore balance to these systems.

Here are some common acupressure techniques that target the twelve major meridians:

Press and Release Technique

This technique involves applying firm pressure to an acupressure point for a few seconds, and then releasing the pressure for a few seconds before repeating. This technique can be used to promote relaxation and relieve tension in the body.

For example, to target the Lung meridian, the practitioner may apply pressure to the Lung 1 point located on the outer edge of the chest, just below the collarbone.

Circular Technique

The circular technique involves applying pressure to an acupressure point in a circular motion using the fingertips or thumb. This technique can be used to stimulate blood flow and promote healing in the body.

For example, to target the Spleen meridian, the practitioner may apply circular pressure to the Spleen 6 point located on the inner side of the leg, about three finger widths above the ankle bone.

Kneading Technique

The kneading technique involves applying pressure to an acupressure point using a kneading motion with the fingertips or thumb. This technique can be used to relieve tension and promote relaxation in the body.

For example, to target the Stomach meridian, the practitioner may apply kneading pressure to the Stomach 36 point located on the lower leg, about four finger widths below the kneecap.

Tapping Technique

The tapping technique involves tapping an acupressure point with the fingertips or knuckles. This technique can be used to stimulate blood flow and promote healing in the body.

For example, to target the Liver meridian, the practitioner may tap the Liver 3 point located on the top of the foot, in the depression between the big toe and the second toe.

Holding Technique

The holding technique involves applying firm pressure to an acupressure point and holding it for a period of time, typically 30 seconds to a minute. This technique can be used to promote relaxation and relieve tension in the body.

For example, to target the Heart meridian, the practitioner may apply pressure to the Heart 7 point located on the wrist, in the depression on the palm side of the wrist below the base of the thumb.

Acupressure can be performed by a trained practitioner or self-administered at home. When performing acupressure on yourself, it's important to locate the correct acupressure points and apply pressure with the appropriate technique.

In addition to the above techniques, acupressure can also be performed using various tools, such as acupressure mats, rollers, and balls. These tools can help target specific areas of the body and provide deeper pressure than finger or hand techniques.

Introduction to Acupressure

Acupressure is a form of traditional Chinese medicine (TCM) that has been used for thousands of years to promote health and well-being. It involves applying pressure to specific points on the body to stimulate the body's natural healing abilities and restore balance to the body's energy flow, also known as Qi.

In TCM, the body is seen as a complex system of interconnected channels or meridians, through which Qi flows. There are twelve major meridians in the body, each corresponding to specific organs and systems, and by applying pressure to the appropriate points along these meridians, acupressure can help restore balance to the body and promote optimal health.

Acupressure is based on the same principles as acupuncture, but instead of using needles, pressure is applied using the fingers, hands, elbows, or other devices. The pressure can be applied in a variety of ways, including rubbing, kneading, tapping, or holding.

One of the key benefits of acupressure is its ability to stimulate the body's natural healing mechanisms. By targeting specific points along the body's meridians, acupressure can help increase blood flow, promote the flow of Qi, and release tension and stress in the body.

Acupressure can be used to treat a wide range of conditions, including pain, stress, anxiety, depression, digestive disorders, and respiratory problems. It can also be used to promote relaxation and improve overall well-being.

Here are some of the benefits of acupressure and how it relates to the twelve major meridians:

The Lung Meridian

The Lung meridian runs from the chest to the thumb and is associated with the respiratory system. By applying pressure to specific points along the Lung meridian, acupressure can help relieve coughing, asthma, and other respiratory conditions.

The Large Intestine Meridian

The Large Intestine meridian runs from the index finger to the nose and is associated with the digestive system. By applying pressure to specific points along the Large Intestine meridian, acupressure can help relieve constipation, diarrhea, and other digestive disorders.

The Stomach Meridian

The Stomach meridian runs from the face to the foot and is associated with the digestive system. By applying pressure to specific points along the Stomach meridian, acupressure can help relieve nausea, vomiting, and other digestive disorders.

The Spleen Meridian

The Spleen meridian runs from the foot to the chest and is associated with the digestive and immune systems. By applying pressure to specific points along the Spleen meridian, acupressure can help boost the immune system and improve digestion.

The Heart Meridian

The Heart meridian runs from the chest to the pinky finger and is associated with the cardiovascular system. By applying pressure to specific points along the Heart meridian, acupressure can help regulate heart rate and blood pressure, and improve circulation.

The Small Intestine Meridian

The Small Intestine meridian runs from the hand to the face and is associated with the digestive system. By applying pressure to specific points along the Small Intestine meridian, acupressure can help relieve bloating, abdominal pain, and other digestive disorders.

The Bladder Meridian

The Bladder meridian runs from the head to the foot and is associated with the urinary system. By applying pressure to specific points along the Bladder meridian, acupressure can help relieve urinary problems, such as frequent urination and incontinence.

How to Apply Acupressure on Meridian Points

Acupressure is a form of traditional Chinese medicine that involves applying pressure to specific points on the body to stimulate healing and restore balance to the body's energy flow, also known as Qi. By applying pressure to specific points along the body's twelve major meridians, acupressure can help relieve pain, reduce stress, and promote overall well-being.

Here are some steps on how to apply acupressure on meridian points:

Locate the Meridian Points

The first step is to locate the meridian points on the body. The twelve major meridians run throughout the body and are associated with specific organs and systems. Each meridian has multiple points, so it's important to identify the specific point you want to target.

There are many resources available, such as books or websites, that provide diagrams of the meridian points. You can also consult with a licensed acupuncturist or acupressure practitioner for guidance on identifying the correct points.

Apply Pressure

Once you have located the meridian point, use your fingers or a tool to apply pressure to the point. The amount of pressure you apply will depend on the sensitivity of the area and your own comfort level. Start with gentle pressure and gradually increase the pressure as needed.

You can apply pressure using a variety of techniques, such as rubbing, kneading, tapping, or holding. It's important to listen to your body and adjust the pressure as needed to avoid causing pain or discomfort.

Hold the Point

After applying pressure to the point, hold the point for a few seconds or minutes. This allows the body to fully absorb the benefits of the pressure and can help promote relaxation and relieve tension in the area.

Some acupressure points may be more sensitive than others, and holding the point for too long or applying too much pressure can cause discomfort or pain. It's important to pay attention to your body and adjust the pressure or duration as needed.

Repeat as Needed

Acupressure can be done on a regular basis to help maintain balance and promote overall well-being. You can repeat the process on the same meridian point multiple times throughout the day or week, or you can target different meridian points based on your specific needs.

It's important to note that acupressure is not a substitute for medical treatment and should not be used to diagnose or treat a medical condition. If you have a medical condition or are experiencing severe pain or discomfort, it's important to consult with a healthcare provider before attempting acupressure.

Here are some examples of how to apply acupressure on specific meridian points:

Lung Meridian Point

The Lung meridian point is located on the outside of the upper arm, about three finger widths below the shoulder joint. To apply acupressure to this point, use your fingers or a tool to apply pressure to the point for a few seconds or minutes.

This point can help relieve respiratory problems, such as coughing and asthma.

Stomach Meridian Point

The Stomach meridian point is located on the front of the leg, about four finger widths below the kneecap. To apply acupressure to this point, use your fingers or a tool to apply pressure to the point for a few seconds or minutes.

This point can help relieve digestive problems, such as nausea and vomiting.

Spleen Meridian Point

The Spleen meridian point is located on the inside of the lower leg, about four finger widths above the ankle bone. To apply acupressure to this point, use your fingers or a tool to apply pressure to the point for a few seconds or minutes.

Acupuncture and Meridians

Acupuncture is a form of traditional Chinese medicine that involves the insertion of fine needles into specific points along the body's twelve major meridians to stimulate healing and restore balance to the body's energy flow, also known as Qi. The concept of meridians is central to acupuncture, as each meridian is associated with specific organs and systems in the body. Below we will explore the relationship between acupuncture and the twelve major meridians.

The Twelve Major Meridians

The twelve major meridians run throughout the body and are associated with specific organs and systems. Each meridian has multiple points that can be stimulated with acupuncture needles to promote healing and balance.

Here is a brief overview of the twelve major meridians and their associated organs/systems:

Lung Meridian - Associated with the lungs and respiratory system.

Large Intestine Meridian - Associated with the large intestine and digestive system.

Stomach Meridian - Associated with the stomach and digestive system.

Spleen Meridian - Associated with the spleen and immune system.

Heart Meridian - Associated with the heart and circulatory system.

Small Intestine Meridian - Associated with the small intestine and digestive system.

Bladder Meridian - Associated with the bladder and urinary system.

Kidney Meridian - Associated with the kidneys and urinary system.

Pericardium Meridian - Associated with the heart and circulatory system.

Triple Warmer Meridian - Associated with the endocrine system and metabolism.

Gallbladder Meridian - Associated with the gallbladder and digestive system.

Liver Meridian - Associated with the liver and digestive system.

Acupuncture and Meridians

Acupuncture involves the insertion of fine needles into specific points along the body's meridians to stimulate healing and restore balance to the body's energy flow. By stimulating these points, acupuncture can help relieve pain, reduce stress, and promote overall well-being.

Acupuncture needles are inserted into specific points along the meridian, known as acupuncture points. Each acupuncture point is associated with a specific meridian and organ/system in the body. By targeting specific acupuncture points along a meridian, an acupuncturist can help restore balance and promote healing in the associated organ/system.

For example, the Lung meridian is associated with the lungs and respiratory system. By targeting acupuncture points along the Lung meridian, an acupuncturist can help relieve respiratory problems, such as coughing and asthma.

The needles used in acupuncture are very thin and are inserted at varying depths, depending on the location of the acupuncture point and the individual's needs. The needles may be left in place for several minutes or longer, depending on the treatment plan.

Acupuncture is a safe and effective form of complementary and alternative medicine. It is often used in conjunction with other forms of healthcare, such as Western medicine, to help promote healing and overall well-being.

Introduction to Acupuncture

Acupuncture is a traditional Chinese medicine technique that has been practiced for thousands of years. It involves the insertion of fine needles into specific points on the body known as acupuncture points, which are connected to the body's twelve major meridians. These meridians are pathways that carry energy, or Qi, throughout the body. Below we will explore the history, principles, and techniques of acupuncture.

History of Acupuncture

Acupuncture has a long and rich history, dating back over 2,500 years to ancient China. The practice is based on the concept of Qi, which is the vital energy that flows throughout the body. According to traditional Chinese medicine, Qi flows through the body along pathways known as meridians.

The practice of acupuncture was first documented in the Huangdi Neijing, a Chinese medical text that dates back to the 2nd century BCE. The text describes the use of needles to stimulate specific points along the meridians to promote healing and relieve pain.

Acupuncture was introduced to the Western world in the 17th century by Jesuit missionaries in China. However, it wasn't until the 20th century that acupuncture gained widespread popularity in the West.

Principles of Acupuncture

Acupuncture is based on the principle that the body has a natural ability to heal itself. The goal of acupuncture is to stimulate the body's natural healing mechanisms by restoring balance to the flow of Qi along the body's meridians.

Acupuncture points are located along the meridians, and each point is associated with specific organs and systems in the body. By stimulating these points, acupuncture can help to restore balance and promote healing in the associated organs and systems.

The body's twelve major meridians are divided into six Yin and six Yang meridians. Yin meridians are associated with the internal organs, while Yang meridians are associated with the external body structures. The balance between Yin and Yang is essential for optimal health, and acupuncture aims to restore this balance.

Acupuncture Techniques

Acupuncture involves the insertion of fine, sterile needles into specific acupuncture points on the body. The needles are left in place for anywhere from a few minutes to an hour, depending on the treatment plan.

The sensation of acupuncture varies from person to person. Some people report feeling a slight pinch or tingling sensation when the needle is inserted, while others report feeling nothing at all.

Acupuncture can be used to treat a wide range of conditions, including:

Pain

Headaches and migraines

Digestive problems

Anxiety and depression

Insomnia

Infertility

Allergies and asthma

Menstrual and menopausal symptoms

Acupuncture is generally considered safe when performed by a licensed practitioner using sterile needles. However, as with any medical treatment, there are some risks associated with acupuncture, such as bleeding, bruising, and infection.

How Acupuncture Works with the Meridian System

Acupuncture is an ancient healing art that has been used for thousands of years to treat a variety of health conditions. It involves the insertion of thin, sterile needles into specific points on the body known as acupoints, which are located along the body's meridian pathways. In traditional Chinese medicine (TCM), the meridian system is believed to be the body's energy network, through which vital energy or Qi flows.

The concept of Qi, which is often translated as vital energy, is central to TCM theory. According to TCM, Qi flows through the body along twelve main meridian pathways, each of which is associated with a particular organ system. The meridian system is considered to be a complex network that connects all parts of the body, including the organs, tissues, and cells.

In acupuncture, the practitioner carefully selects acupoints along the meridian pathway to address the specific health concern of the patient. The needles are inserted into the acupoints and left in place for a period of time, usually around 20-30 minutes. During this time, the patient may feel a sensation of heaviness, warmth, or tingling in the area surrounding the needle.

The theory behind acupuncture is that the insertion of the needles into the acupoints stimulates the flow of Qi along the meridian pathway. This is believed to restore balance and harmony to the body, promoting the body's natural healing abilities. In TCM theory, illness is seen as a disruption in the flow of Qi, which can be caused by a variety of factors such as stress, poor diet, and environmental toxins.

Acupuncture is often used to treat a wide range of health conditions, including pain, digestive disorders, respiratory conditions, and emotional imbalances. It is also commonly used as a complementary therapy to conventional medical treatments such as chemotherapy and surgery.

The effectiveness of acupuncture has been the subject of much scientific research in recent years. While the exact mechanisms of how acupuncture works are not yet fully understood, studies have shown that it can have a significant impact on the body's pain response, immune system, and hormonal balance.

Acupuncture is a safe and non-invasive therapy that is generally well-tolerated by most people. However, it is important to seek out a qualified and licensed acupuncturist who has received extensive training in the meridian system and the practice of acupuncture.

Moxibustion and Meridians

Moxibustion is a traditional Chinese medicine therapy that involves the burning of dried mugwort (Artemisia vulgaris) on or near acupoints on the body. This therapy is often used in conjunction with acupuncture to stimulate the flow of Qi, or vital energy, along the body's meridian pathways.

In traditional Chinese medicine theory, the meridian system is the network of pathways through which Qi flows. The twelve major meridians correspond to specific organs and organ systems in the body and are believed to be connected to the body's overall health and wellbeing.

Moxibustion is thought to work by stimulating the flow of Qi along the meridian pathways, promoting the body's natural healing response. When mugwort is burned, it produces a heat that penetrates the skin and stimulates the acupoints and meridians. This can improve circulation and stimulate the immune system, helping to promote healing and balance within the body.

Moxibustion is commonly used to treat a variety of health conditions, including digestive disorders, menstrual cramps, arthritis, and asthma. It can also be used to help boost the immune system and improve overall health and wellbeing.

There are two main types of moxibustion: direct and indirect. Direct moxibustion involves placing a small amount of moxa directly on the skin and burning it until it is warm. Indirect moxibustion involves the use of a moxa stick or cone that is held near the skin, producing a heat that penetrates the acupoints and meridians.

In addition to its therapeutic benefits, moxibustion is also considered to be a relaxing and calming therapy. Many people find the warm sensation of moxibustion to be comforting and soothing, making it a popular therapy for stress relief and relaxation.

Moxibustion is generally considered to be safe when performed by a qualified practitioner. However, it is important to note that moxibustion should not be used on certain areas of the body, such as the face or genitals, and should not be used on individuals with certain medical conditions, such as pregnancy or certain skin conditions.

Introduction to Moxibustion

Moxibustion is an ancient Chinese therapy that has been used for thousands of years to promote healing, relieve pain, and prevent disease. It is a form of heat therapy that involves burning dried mugwort (Artemisia vulgaris) and placing it on or near specific acupuncture points on the body. Moxibustion is an important part of traditional Chinese medicine and is often used in conjunction with acupuncture to enhance its therapeutic effects.

History of Moxibustion

The history of moxibustion can be traced back to the earliest records of traditional Chinese medicine. The earliest known reference to moxibustion dates back to the Huangdi Neijing (The Yellow Emperor's Classic of Internal Medicine), a medical text that was written over 2,000 years ago. This text describes the use of moxibustion to treat a wide range of conditions, including colds, flu, arthritis, and digestive disorders.

Over the centuries, moxibustion has continued to be an important part of traditional Chinese medicine. It is now widely used in many parts of the world, including Japan, Korea, and Vietnam.

Types of Moxibustion

There are two main types of moxibustion: direct and indirect.

Direct moxibustion involves placing a small cone of moxa directly on the skin at an acupuncture point. The moxa is then lit and allowed to burn until it is extinguished or removed. Direct moxibustion is often used to treat acute conditions and is thought to have a stronger therapeutic effect.

Indirect moxibustion involves placing a small amount of moxa on the end of an acupuncture needle, which is then inserted into the skin. The moxa is then lit and allowed to burn until it is extinguished or removed. Indirect moxibustion is often used to treat chronic conditions and is thought to have a gentler therapeutic effect.

Benefits of Moxibustion

Moxibustion is believed to have a number of benefits for the body, including:

Promoting healing: The heat from the moxa is believed to increase circulation, stimulate the immune system, and promote the flow of qi (energy) throughout the body. This can help to promote healing and reduce inflammation.

Relieving pain: Moxibustion is often used to relieve pain, especially in the joints and muscles. The heat from the moxa is believed to stimulate the release of natural pain-relieving chemicals in the body.

Improving digestion: Moxibustion is often used to treat digestive disorders, such as bloating, nausea, and diarrhea. The heat from the moxa is believed to stimulate the digestive system and promote the flow of qi.

Boosting immunity: Moxibustion is believed to stimulate the immune system, which can help to prevent illness and disease.

Regulating menstrual cycles: Moxibustion is often used to treat menstrual disorders, such as irregular periods and cramps. The heat from the moxa is believed to promote the flow of blood and qi in the pelvic region.

How Moxibustion Works with the Meridian System

Moxibustion works with the meridian system in a similar way to acupuncture. The meridians are channels that run throughout the body, carrying qi and other vital substances. When these channels become blocked or imbalanced, illness and disease can result.

The Benefits of Moxibustion on Meridian Health

Moxibustion is a traditional Chinese medicine therapy that involves burning mugwort herb (Artemisia vulgaris) to stimulate acupuncture points or meridians. This therapy has been used for centuries in China, Japan, and Korea to promote healing and prevent illness. The benefits of moxibustion on meridian health are vast and have been proven effective in various studies.

The meridians in traditional Chinese medicine are pathways or channels through which the vital energy (Qi) flows. Qi is believed to be the life force that controls the body's functions, including the organs, tissues, and systems. According to traditional Chinese medicine, the smooth flow of Qi through the meridians is essential for good health. When Qi is blocked or stagnant in the meridians, it can cause disease or illness.

Moxibustion is an effective therapy that helps to unblock and regulate the flow of Qi in the meridians. The heat generated by burning mugwort herb on acupuncture points or meridians helps to increase blood circulation, stimulate the immune system, and promote relaxation. Moxibustion also helps to relieve pain and inflammation, improve digestion, boost energy, and enhance overall health and wellbeing.

One of the benefits of moxibustion on meridian health is its ability to improve the function of the digestive system. In traditional Chinese medicine, the Spleen and Stomach meridians are responsible for the digestion of food and the absorption of nutrients. When these meridians are blocked or deficient, it can lead to poor digestion, bloating, diarrhea, and other digestive problems. Moxibustion on the Spleen and Stomach meridians can help to improve the function of these organs, increase the production of digestive enzymes, and promote the absorption of nutrients.

Moxibustion is also beneficial for the Respiratory meridians, which include the Lung and Large Intestine meridians. The Lung meridian is responsible for the function of the respiratory system, including breathing and oxygenation of the blood. Moxibustion on the Lung meridian can help to improve lung function, increase oxygenation of the blood, and relieve respiratory problems such as asthma, bronchitis, and pneumonia.

The Large Intestine meridian is responsible for the elimination of waste from the body. When this meridian is blocked or stagnant, it can lead to constipation, diarrhea, and other bowel problems. Moxibustion on the Large Intestine meridian can help to stimulate bowel movements, improve digestion, and promote the elimination of waste from the body.

Another benefit of moxibustion on meridian health is its ability to boost the immune system. The immune system is responsible for protecting the body against infections and diseases. When the immune system is weak, the body is more susceptible to illness. Moxibustion on the immune system meridians, including the Spleen, Stomach, and Kidney meridians, can help to boost the immune system, increase the production of white blood cells, and enhance the body's ability to fight infections and diseases.

Moxibustion is also beneficial for the reproductive system meridians, including the Kidney and Liver meridians. The Kidney meridian is responsible for the function of the reproductive system, including fertility and sexual function. Moxibustion on the Kidney meridian can help to improve fertility, regulate menstrual cycles, and relieve symptoms of menopause.

Cupping Therapy and Meridians

Cupping therapy is an ancient healing technique that has been used for thousands of years in traditional Chinese medicine (TCM). The practice involves placing cups made of bamboo, glass, or other materials on the skin to create suction, which is believed to stimulate the flow of qi or energy along the meridians. Below we will explore the relationship between cupping therapy and meridians, and how this therapy can benefit meridian health.

In TCM, meridians are believed to be pathways that carry energy throughout the body. When energy is flowing smoothly through these channels, the body is in a state of balance and health. However, when energy becomes blocked or stagnated, it can lead to pain, illness, and disease. Cupping therapy is one of the many techniques used in TCM to promote the flow of energy along the meridians and restore balance to the body.

During a cupping therapy session, the therapist places cups on the skin, usually on the back, neck, or shoulders. The cups create suction, which pulls the skin and underlying tissues upward into the cup. This suction is thought to increase blood flow, stimulate the lymphatic system, and release tension in the muscles and fascia. In TCM, this is believed to promote the flow of qi along the meridians and restore balance to the body.

There are several ways that cupping therapy can benefit meridian health. First, by increasing blood flow and stimulating the lymphatic system, cupping can help to clear any blockages or stagnation in the meridians. This can help to alleviate pain, reduce inflammation, and improve overall organ function.

Second, cupping therapy can also help to release tension in the muscles and fascia. When muscles are tight or in spasm, they can compress the meridians and impede the flow of energy. By releasing this tension, cupping therapy can help to open up the meridians and promote the free flow of energy throughout the body.

Third, cupping therapy can also be used to tonify or strengthen specific meridians. In TCM, certain meridians are associated with specific organs or body systems. By placing cups on specific points along these meridians, cupping therapy can help to nourish and strengthen these organs or systems, and promote overall health and wellbeing.

There are several different types of cupping therapy that can be used to benefit meridian health. The most common form of cupping is dry cupping, which involves placing cups on the skin and creating suction without using any additional substances. Another form of cupping is wet cupping, which involves creating small incisions in the skin before placing the cups. This allows for the release of small amounts of blood and can help to remove toxins and improve circulation.

Fire cupping is another type of cupping therapy that involves using heat to create suction. In this technique, the therapist will light a small flame inside the cup to create a vacuum before placing it on the skin. This technique is thought to be particularly effective for tonifying or strengthening specific meridians.

Introduction to Cupping Therapy

Cupping therapy is an ancient healing technique that has been used in traditional medicine for thousands of years. It involves the use of cups, which are typically made of glass, plastic, or bamboo, that are placed on the skin to create suction. The suction draws the skin and underlying tissue into the cup, which is believed to stimulate the flow of energy, or Qi, through the body's meridian system.

In traditional Chinese medicine, the meridian system is a network of energy channels that run throughout the body. It is believed that this system plays a vital role in regulating the body's functions and maintaining overall health and well-being. The meridian system is made up of 12 main meridians, which correspond to specific organs and bodily systems.

Cupping therapy is often used to help regulate the flow of Qi through the meridian system. The suction created by the cups is believed to help remove blockages and stimulate the flow of energy through the meridians. This can help to improve circulation, relieve pain and tension, and promote overall health and well-being.

There are several different types of cupping therapy, including dry cupping, wet cupping, and fire cupping. Dry cupping involves placing the cups on the skin without any additional treatment. Wet cupping involves making small incisions in the skin before placing the cups, which allows for the removal of blood and other fluids. Fire cupping involves using a flame to heat the air inside the cup before placing it on the skin, which creates suction.

Cupping therapy is often used to treat a variety of conditions, including musculoskeletal pain, respiratory disorders, digestive issues, and stress-related conditions. It is also commonly used as a form of complementary therapy to support overall health and well-being.

One of the key benefits of cupping therapy is its ability to stimulate the flow of energy through the meridian system. This can help to improve circulation and promote the delivery of oxygen and nutrients to the body's cells and tissues. It can also help to remove blockages and improve the flow of lymphatic fluid, which plays a key role in the body's immune system.

Cupping therapy is also believed to have a number of other benefits, including reducing inflammation, relieving pain and tension, improving digestion, and promoting relaxation and stress relief. It is often used in conjunction with other traditional Chinese medicine therapies, such as acupuncture and herbal medicine, to provide a comprehensive approach to health and wellness.

How Cupping Therapy Affects the Meridian System

Cupping therapy is an ancient healing technique that is often used in Traditional Chinese Medicine (TCM). It involves placing cups on the skin and creating a vacuum to stimulate blood flow and promote healing. Cupping therapy is often used in conjunction with other TCM practices, such as acupuncture and herbal medicine, to promote overall health and wellbeing. Below we will explore how cupping therapy affects the meridian system and how it can promote optimal health.

To understand how cupping therapy affects the meridian system, we must first understand what the meridian system is. The meridian system is a network of channels that flow throughout the body and connect the various organs and tissues. According to TCM, these channels are responsible for the flow of qi (pronounced "chee"), which is the vital life force energy that flows throughout the body. When the flow of qi is disrupted, it can lead to illness and disease.

Cupping therapy works by stimulating blood flow to the affected area, which can help to clear blockages and restore the flow of qi. When the cups are placed on the skin, they create a vacuum that draws the skin and underlying tissues upward, creating a suction effect. This suction effect stimulates blood flow to the area and can help to promote healing.

In TCM, the meridian system is divided into twelve major channels, each of which is associated with a different organ system in the body. These channels are known as the Lung, Large Intestine, Stomach, Spleen, Heart, Small Intestine, Bladder, Kidney, Pericardium, Triple Burner, Gallbladder, and Liver meridians. Each of these meridians has specific acupoints that are associated with them and that can be targeted with cupping therapy.

For example, if someone is experiencing digestive issues, their TCM practitioner may focus on the Stomach and Large Intestine meridians. By placing cups on the acupoints associated with these meridians, they can stimulate blood flow to these areas and promote optimal digestive function. Similarly, if someone is experiencing anxiety or stress, their practitioner may focus on the Heart and Pericardium meridians, as these are associated with emotional wellbeing.

In addition to promoting optimal function of the specific organ systems associated with each meridian, cupping therapy can also have systemic effects on the body. For example, it can help to boost the immune system, improve circulation, and reduce inflammation. By promoting overall health and wellbeing, cupping therapy can help to prevent illness and disease before they occur.

There are several different types of cupping therapy that can be used to stimulate the meridian system. These include:

Dry cupping: This is the most common type of cupping therapy and involves placing cups on the skin and leaving them in place for a set period of time, usually between 5 and 10 minutes.

Wet cupping: This involves making small incisions in the skin before applying the cups. The cups are left in place for a shorter period of time, and the practitioner may use a small amount of suction to remove a small amount of blood from the incision site.

Fire cupping: This involves briefly heating the inside of the cup before applying it to the skin. The heat creates a vacuum that draws the skin and underlying tissues upward.

Massage cupping: This involves applying oil to the skin before using the cups to massage the area. This can help to promote relaxation and reduce muscle tension.

Qigong and Meridian Exercises

Qigong is an ancient Chinese practice that involves gentle movements, breathing exercises, and meditation to improve physical and mental health. The practice of Qigong is rooted in Traditional Chinese Medicine (TCM) and is believed to promote the flow of Qi or vital energy in the body. The concept of Qi is closely related to the Meridian system in TCM, which refers to the network of pathways that run throughout the body, carrying Qi and blood to nourish and maintain the organs and tissues.

In Qigong, the Meridian system plays a crucial role as it is believed to be the key to unlocking the flow of Qi in the body. There are twelve major meridians in the body, each of which is associated with a specific organ system and has a unique set of functions. These meridians are paired, with each pair corresponding to a specific element and representing the interplay between yin and yang energies. Qigong exercises are designed to stimulate and balance the flow of Qi in these meridians, promoting overall health and wellbeing.

One of the main benefits of Qigong is that it can help to improve circulation in the body, which is crucial for the proper functioning of the organs and tissues. When the flow of Qi is disrupted or blocked, it can lead to a variety of health problems such as pain, inflammation, and disease. By practicing Qigong, individuals can promote the smooth flow of Qi throughout the body, helping to reduce the risk of these health problems.

In addition to improving circulation, Qigong can also help to reduce stress and anxiety, improve mental clarity, and promote relaxation. This is because the practice of Qigong involves mindfulness and focused breathing, which can help to calm the mind and reduce tension in the body. By promoting relaxation and reducing stress, Qigong can also help to boost the immune system, which is essential for maintaining good health and preventing illness.

Qigong exercises that focus on the Meridian system are typically designed to target specific organs or organ systems, helping to balance the flow of Qi and restore health to the body. For example, the Lung Meridian is associated with the respiratory system, and Qigong exercises that focus on this meridian can help to improve lung function and reduce the risk of respiratory problems such as asthma and bronchitis. The Spleen Meridian is associated with digestion, and Qigong exercises that stimulate this meridian can help to improve digestion and reduce the risk of digestive problems such as bloating and constipation.

There are many different Qigong exercises that focus on the Meridian system, each with its own unique benefits. Some of the most popular Qigong exercises include the Eight Brocades, the Five Animal Frolics, and the Six Healing Sounds. These exercises can be practiced individually or as part of a larger Qigong routine, and can be adapted to suit the needs of individuals at any age or fitness level.

Introduction to Qigong

Qigong is a traditional Chinese practice that involves a combination of gentle movements, deep breathing techniques, and mental focus to promote health and wellbeing. The word Qigong is composed of two Chinese characters - Qi, meaning vital energy or life force, and Gong, meaning practice or cultivation. The practice of Qigong is believed to enhance the flow of Qi throughout the body, promoting a balance of yin and yang energy and strengthening the meridian system.

The origins of Qigong can be traced back to ancient China, where it was developed as a component of traditional Chinese medicine. Qigong was traditionally used to treat a variety of health conditions, including respiratory problems, cardiovascular disease, digestive disorders, and mental health issues.

Qigong is based on the principle that Qi flows throughout the body via a network of channels known as meridians. According to traditional Chinese medicine, there are twelve main meridians that run through the body, each of which is associated with specific organs and functions. These meridians are thought to be interconnected and dependent on each other, forming a complex network that regulates the flow of Qi and maintains the balance of yin and yang energy.

In Qigong practice, practitioners use various techniques to stimulate the flow of Qi and balance the meridian system. These techniques include movements, breathing exercises, meditation, and visualization. Some Qigong forms involve slow, fluid movements that mimic the movements of animals or nature, while others focus on specific postures or breathing patterns.

One of the key principles of Qigong is the idea of "Zhuang Yuan," or "posture power." This concept emphasizes the importance of maintaining proper alignment and relaxation of the body to facilitate the flow of Qi. By practicing Qigong regularly, individuals can strengthen their meridian system, balance their yin and yang energy, and promote overall health and wellbeing.

Research has shown that Qigong can have a wide range of benefits for physical and mental health. Studies have found that regular Qigong practice can reduce stress and anxiety, improve immune function, and lower blood pressure and cholesterol levels. Qigong has also been shown to improve balance and coordination, relieve chronic pain, and enhance overall quality of life.

In addition to its health benefits, Qigong is also considered a spiritual practice in Chinese culture. Many Qigong practitioners incorporate meditation and visualization techniques to cultivate a sense of inner peace and harmony.

Meridian Exercises for Health and Balance

Meridian exercises are a form of qigong, a traditional Chinese practice that involves a combination of physical movement, meditation, and breath control. These exercises focus on stimulating the flow of qi (pronounced "chee"), the vital energy that flows through the meridians or energy pathways in the body. Meridian exercises are simple and easy to perform, and can be practiced by people of all ages and fitness levels. Below we will explore some of the most effective meridian exercises for health and balance.

The Inner Smile Meditation

The Inner Smile meditation is a simple yet powerful technique that can help to release tension and negativity from the body and mind. It involves focusing on different parts of the body and sending them positive energy and love. This meditation can be performed in a seated or standing position.

To begin, take a deep breath and relax your body. Close your eyes and bring your awareness to your heart center. Imagine a beautiful, warm, smiling light radiating from your heart, filling your entire body with warmth and positivity. As you inhale, imagine this light expanding and filling your entire body. As you exhale, imagine any negativity, tension, or pain leaving your body and being replaced by the warm, healing light.

Next, focus on each organ in the body and visualize it being filled with positive energy. Begin with the lungs, then move on to the liver, spleen, pancreas, kidneys, heart, and brain. Finally, focus on the meridians that connect these organs, visualizing them as glowing pathways of light that connect and nourish the body.

The Eight Pieces of Brocade

The Eight Pieces of Brocade, also known as Ba Duan Jin, is a set of eight simple movements that can help to improve the flow of qi and stimulate the major meridians in the body. These exercises can be performed in a seated or standing position.

To begin, stand with your feet shoulder-width apart and your arms at your sides. Inhale deeply, raising your arms to shoulder height, with your palms facing up. Exhale and slowly lower your arms to your sides. Repeat this movement five times.

Next, inhale and raise your arms above your head, with your palms facing each other. Exhale and lower your arms to your sides. Repeat this movement five times.

Next, inhale and raise your arms above your head, with your palms facing up. Exhale and slowly bend forward, reaching for your toes. Inhale and slowly rise back up, raising your arms above your head. Exhale and lower your arms to your sides. Repeat this movement five times.

Continue with the remaining movements, which include rotating the waist, extending the arms and legs, and twisting the torso.

The Dragon and Tiger Qigong

The Dragon and Tiger Qigong is a set of movements that focus on stretching and opening the major meridians in the body. These exercises can be performed in a standing or seated position.

To begin, stand with your feet shoulder-width apart and your arms at your sides. Inhale deeply, raising your arms to shoulder height, with your palms facing up. Exhale and slowly lower your arms to your sides. Repeat this movement three times.

Next, inhale and raise your arms above your head, with your palms facing each other. Exhale and slowly lower your arms to your sides. Repeat this movement three times.

Next, inhale and raise your arms above your head, with your palms facing up. Exhale and slowly bend forward, reaching for your toes. Inhale and slowly rise back up, raising your arms above your head. Exhale and lower your arms to your sides. Repeat this movement three times.

Meridian Meditation Techniques

Meridian meditation is a practice that involves using breath, visualization, and intention to stimulate the flow of energy through the body's meridian system. The meridian system is a complex network of energy pathways that run throughout the body and are essential to traditional Chinese medicine. Below we will explore meridian meditation techniques and how they can help promote health and balance.

The meridian system is composed of 12 major meridians and 8 extraordinary meridians that connect the body's organs and tissues. Each meridian is associated with a specific organ system and has a unique pattern of energy flow. Traditional Chinese medicine teaches that when the energy flow in the meridians is blocked or disrupted, illness and disease can occur.

Meridian meditation is a practice that can help stimulate the flow of energy through the meridians, promoting health and balance. One common technique used in meridian meditation is to focus on the breath. By taking slow, deep breaths, we can help calm the mind and body, which can improve the flow of energy through the meridians.

Another technique used in meridian meditation is visualization. By visualizing the flow of energy through the meridians, we can help stimulate the flow of energy and clear any blockages that may be present. This can be done by imagining a stream of light or energy flowing through each meridian, from the starting point to the endpoint.

Intention is also an essential component of meridian meditation. By setting an intention for the meditation practice, we can help direct the flow of energy through the meridians to specific areas of the body. For example, if we are experiencing pain or discomfort in a particular area, we can set the intention to direct the flow of energy to that area to help promote healing.

There are many meridian meditation techniques that can be used to promote health and balance in the body. One such technique is the Five Elements Meditation, which is based on the principles of traditional Chinese medicine. This meditation involves focusing on the five elements – wood, fire, earth, metal, and water – and their associated meridians.

To perform the Five Elements Meditation, start by finding a quiet, comfortable space where you can sit or lie down. Close your eyes and take several slow, deep breaths to help calm your mind and body. Next, visualize each element in turn, starting with wood. As you focus on each element, imagine the corresponding meridian and visualize the flow of energy through that meridian.

For example, when focusing on the wood element, visualize the liver meridian and imagine a stream of energy flowing smoothly through that meridian. Repeat this process for each element and associated meridian, taking as much time as you need to fully focus on each one.

Another meridian meditation technique is the Meridian Tracing Meditation, which involves tracing the meridians with your hands while visualizing the flow of energy through the meridians. To perform this meditation, start by finding a quiet, comfortable space where you can sit or stand. Begin by placing your hands on your belly and taking several slow, deep breaths to help calm your mind and body.

Next, slowly trace the meridians with your hands, starting with the lung meridian and working your way through each meridian in turn. As you trace each meridian, visualize the flow of energy through that meridian, imagining any blockages being cleared and the flow of energy becoming smooth and even.

The Importance of Meditation

Meditation is an ancient practice that has been used for thousands of years to promote physical, mental, and emotional health. It involves training the mind to focus and achieve a state of calmness and relaxation. Meditation has been linked to a variety of health benefits, including reducing stress and anxiety, improving sleep quality, increasing attention and focus, and enhancing overall well-being. In the context of Traditional Chinese Medicine (TCM), meditation is an important tool for promoting meridian health and balance.

TCM is a system of medicine that has been used in China for thousands of years. It views the body as a complex network of meridians, or channels, through which vital energy (Qi) flows. When the flow of Qi is disrupted or blocked, it can lead to imbalances and disease. TCM practitioners use a variety of techniques to restore the flow of Qi and promote balance in the body, including acupuncture, acupressure, herbal medicine, and meditation.

Meditation is considered an important component of TCM because it helps to promote the flow of Qi and enhance the function of the meridians. There are several different types of meditation that can be used to achieve this goal. One popular type of meditation in TCM is known as "Qigong" or "Chi Kung". Qigong is a practice that involves a combination of meditation, breathing techniques, and gentle movements designed to promote balance and harmony in the body. It is often used as a form of preventive medicine to promote overall health and well-being.

In TCM, it is believed that each meridian is associated with a different organ system in the body. By practicing Qigong or other meditation techniques, one can focus on specific meridians to promote the flow of Qi to the associated organs. For example, practicing meditation techniques that focus on the Lung meridian can help to promote healthy respiratory function, while focusing on the Liver meridian can help to promote healthy digestion and detoxification.

Meditation is also believed to have a direct effect on the nervous system, which is closely linked to the meridian system in TCM. By promoting a state of calmness and relaxation, meditation can help to reduce stress and anxiety, which are common factors that can disrupt the flow of Qi and lead to imbalances in the body. In addition, meditation has been shown to increase the production of endorphins, which are natural chemicals in the body that promote feelings of happiness and well-being.

Another benefit of meditation in TCM is that it can help to improve the mind-body connection. By focusing on the meridians and the flow of Qi through the body, meditation can help to enhance awareness of the body and promote a sense of inner peace and balance. This can be particularly helpful for individuals who suffer from chronic pain or other health conditions that can disrupt the mind-body connection.

Meridian-Based Meditation Practices

Meridian-based meditation practices are a powerful way to promote health and balance in the body and mind. In traditional Chinese medicine, the meridian system is considered the pathway through which vital energy or qi flows. These pathways connect to various organs and functions in the body, and are thought to be intimately connected to our physical, emotional, and mental well-being. By meditating on these meridians and using specific techniques to enhance their function, we can tap into this powerful system to promote health and vitality.

One of the most important concepts in meridian-based meditation is the idea of balance. In Chinese medicine, health is considered a state of balance between yin and yang energies. Yin energy is associated with coolness, quiet, and inwardness, while yang energy is associated with warmth, activity, and outward expression. When these energies are in balance, we experience a sense of well-being and vitality. However, when one energy is in excess or deficient, we may experience various physical or emotional symptoms.

To balance these energies and promote health, meridian-based meditation practices often focus on specific meridians or pairs of meridians that are associated with different organs and functions in the body. For example, the lung meridian is associated with the respiratory system and is believed to be important for the immune system, while the liver meridian is associated with the digestive system and is thought to be important for emotional well-being.

There are many different techniques that can be used in meridian-based meditation, but one common approach is to focus on specific acupoints along the meridians. Acupoints are specific locations along the meridians where the energy is believed to be particularly strong or accessible. By meditating on these points and using specific breathing or visualization techniques, we can enhance the flow of energy through the meridian and promote balance in the associated organ or function.

Another common technique in meridian-based meditation is to use sound or vibration to stimulate the meridian. In Chinese medicine, each meridian is associated with a specific sound or vibration, and by focusing on these sounds or using tools like tuning forks or singing bowls, we can enhance the flow of energy through the meridian and promote balance.

One important aspect of meridian-based meditation is that it is often combined with other holistic practices like acupuncture, herbal medicine, or dietary therapy. By using multiple modalities to address imbalances in the body, we can create a comprehensive approach to health that addresses the root causes of disease rather than just treating symptoms.

There are many different types of meridian-based meditation practices, but some of the most common include qigong, tai chi, and yoga. Qigong is a Chinese practice that involves gentle movements, breathing exercises, and meditation to enhance the flow of qi through the meridians. Tai chi is another Chinese practice that involves slow, flowing movements and meditation to promote balance and relaxation. Yoga is an ancient Indian practice that combines physical postures, breathing exercises, and meditation to promote health and well-being.

Regardless of the specific practice, meridian-based meditation is a powerful tool for promoting health and balance in the body and mind. By tapping into the power of the meridian system and using specific techniques to enhance its function, we can create a deep sense of peace, relaxation, and vitality that can enhance all aspects of our lives. Whether you are dealing with physical symptoms or emotional stress, meridian-based meditation practices offer a gentle and effective way to promote health and well-being from the inside out.

The Role of Nutrition in Meridian Health

The concept of meridians in Traditional Chinese Medicine (TCM) suggests that energy flows through the body in specific pathways, and that these pathways can affect one's health and wellbeing. The twelve major meridians are the channels through which energy, or qi, flows in the body. Nutrition plays a critical role in maintaining the health of these meridians and the overall balance of qi in the body.

According to TCM, each meridian is associated with a specific organ or system in the body, and is linked to specific symptoms and health conditions when its energy flow is disrupted or blocked. Proper nutrition is essential to maintaining the balance and flow of qi in each meridian.

The Spleen meridian, for example, is responsible for transforming food into qi and blood, and is closely related to the digestive system. In TCM, the Spleen is also associated with the emotion of worry, and is said to be weakened by excessive worry or overthinking. A diet that is rich in easily digestible, nutrient-dense foods such as whole grains, legumes, and vegetables can help support the Spleen meridian and promote healthy digestion. On the other hand, consuming too much cold or raw food can weaken the Spleen and disrupt its function.

The Liver meridian is responsible for the smooth flow of qi throughout the body, and is associated with the emotion of anger. A diet that is high in healthy fats, such as those found in nuts, seeds, and fatty fish, can help support the function of the Liver meridian. Conversely, a diet that is high in processed foods, alcohol, and unhealthy fats can weaken the Liver meridian and contribute to the development of health issues such as headaches, menstrual cramps, and emotional instability.

The Kidney meridian is responsible for the growth, development, and reproduction of the body, and is associated with the emotion of fear. A diet that is high in protein and minerals, such as those found in meat, fish, and bone broth, can help support the function of the Kidney meridian. On the other hand, a diet that is high in sugar, caffeine, and processed foods can weaken the Kidney meridian and contribute to health issues such as low back pain, urinary problems, and fatigue.

In addition to eating a healthy, balanced diet, there are several other nutrition-related practices that can help support the health of the meridians. For example, drinking warm liquids such as tea or bone broth can help stimulate the flow of qi, while avoiding cold or iced beverages can help prevent stagnation. Chewing food thoroughly and eating in a calm and relaxed environment can also help support healthy digestion and promote the flow of qi.

In TCM, certain foods are believed to have specific properties that can help support the function of specific meridians. For example, bitter foods such as dark leafy greens and bitter melon are said to stimulate the flow of qi in the Liver meridian, while sour foods such as vinegar and lemon can help tonify the Spleen meridian. Sweet foods such as honey and dates are believed to nourish the Heart meridian, while pungent foods such as ginger and garlic can help promote the flow of qi in the Lung meridian.

The Importance of a Balanced Diet

The concept of a balanced diet has been around for centuries, and it remains as relevant today as it was in the past. A balanced diet is one that provides the body with all the essential nutrients in the right proportions. In the context of meridian health, a balanced diet is even more important because the meridians are responsible for the flow of energy through the body. The foods we eat can either help or hinder this flow, so it is crucial to understand the relationship between nutrition and meridian health.

The twelve major meridians of Traditional Chinese Medicine (TCM) are intimately connected to the organs of the body, and each meridian has specific nutritional requirements to function optimally. The concept of yin and yang is also essential in the context of nutrition and meridian health. In TCM, yin and yang are the two opposing forces that must be in balance for optimal health. Foods can be classified as either yin or yang, depending on their energetic properties. A balanced diet includes foods that are both yin and yang, so the body can maintain a state of balance.

Let's take a closer look at some of the meridians and their corresponding nutritional needs.

The Spleen Meridian

The Spleen Meridian is responsible for the digestion and absorption of nutrients, making it crucial for maintaining optimal nutritional health. The spleen is also responsible for producing blood, so iron-rich foods are essential for the health of this meridian. Foods that are beneficial for the spleen meridian include whole grains, legumes, root vegetables, and leafy greens.

The Liver Meridian

The Liver Meridian is responsible for detoxifying the body, so it requires a diet that is low in toxins. Foods that are high in antioxidants, such as berries and leafy greens, are beneficial for the liver meridian. Healthy fats, such as those found in avocado and olive oil, are also essential for liver health.

The Kidney Meridian

The Kidney Meridian is responsible for the health of the urinary system, so hydration is crucial for this meridian. Foods that are high in water content, such as fruits and vegetables, are beneficial for the kidney meridian. Foods that are high in sodium and caffeine, such as processed foods and coffee, should be avoided, as they can dehydrate the body.

The Heart Meridian

The Heart Meridian is responsible for the circulatory system, making it crucial for cardiovascular health. Foods that are high in omega-3 fatty acids, such as fatty fish and flaxseeds, are beneficial for the heart meridian. Foods that are high in saturated fats, such as processed meats and fried foods, should be avoided.

The Stomach Meridian

The Stomach Meridian is responsible for the digestion of food, making it crucial for digestive health. Foods that are easy to digest, such as cooked vegetables and lean proteins, are beneficial for the stomach meridian. Foods that are high in sugar and fat, such as processed snacks and desserts, should be avoided, as they can disrupt the digestive system.

In addition to eating a balanced diet, it is also essential to pay attention to how you eat. In TCM, it is recommended to eat slowly and mindfully, chewing each bite thoroughly to aid in digestion. Eating in a relaxed and stress-free environment is also beneficial for meridian health.

Foods That Support Meridian Health

Foods play a vital role in supporting the health of the meridians, which are pathways of energy flow in the body according to traditional Chinese medicine. Each meridian is associated with specific organs and bodily functions, and the food we eat can affect their overall health and balance. Below we will discuss foods that support meridian health and help maintain balance in the body.

The Lung Meridian

The Lung Meridian is associated with the respiratory system and is responsible for the intake of oxygen and the removal of carbon dioxide from the body. Foods that support Lung Meridian health include pears, mushrooms, radishes, and white-colored foods such as cauliflower, turnips, and onions. These foods help to nourish the lungs and support the immune system.

The Large Intestine Meridian

The Large Intestine Meridian is responsible for the elimination of waste from the body. Foods that support Large Intestine Meridian health include fiber-rich foods such as whole grains, fruits, and vegetables. These foods help to regulate bowel movements and prevent constipation.

The Stomach Meridian

The Stomach Meridian is responsible for the digestion of food and the absorption of nutrients. Foods that support Stomach Meridian health include warm, cooked foods such as soups, stews, and steamed vegetables. These foods are easy to digest and help to support the digestive system.

The Spleen Meridian

The Spleen Meridian is responsible for the transformation of food into energy and the distribution of nutrients throughout the body. Foods that support Spleen Meridian health include whole grains, legumes, and root vegetables. These foods are high in complex carbohydrates and provide sustained energy throughout the day.

The Heart Meridian

The Heart Meridian is associated with the cardiovascular system and is responsible for the circulation of blood and oxygen throughout the body. Foods that support Heart Meridian health include dark leafy greens, beets, and berries. These foods are high in antioxidants and help to support the cardiovascular system.

The Small Intestine Meridian

The Small Intestine Meridian is responsible for the digestion and absorption of nutrients from food. Foods that support Small Intestine Meridian health include probiotic-rich foods such as yogurt, kefir, and fermented vegetables. These foods help to support a healthy gut microbiome and improve nutrient absorption.

The Bladder Meridian

The Bladder Meridian is responsible for the elimination of waste and excess fluids from the body. Foods that support Bladder Meridian health include diuretic foods such as cucumber, celery, and watermelon. These foods help to reduce fluid retention and promote healthy urinary function.

The Kidney Meridian

The Kidney Meridian is associated with the urinary system and is responsible for the filtration of waste from the blood. Foods that support Kidney Meridian health include kidney beans, black beans, and seaweed. These foods are high in minerals such as potassium and magnesium, which are essential for healthy kidney function.

The Pericardium Meridian

The Pericardium Meridian is associated with the cardiovascular system and is responsible for the regulation of blood pressure and heart rate. Foods that support Pericardium Meridian health include omega-3 rich foods such as fatty fish, nuts, and seeds. These foods help to reduce inflammation and support cardiovascular health.

The Triple Warmer Meridian

The Triple Warmer Meridian is associated with the endocrine system and is responsible for the regulation of hormones in the body. Foods that support Triple Warmer Meridian health include cruciferous vegetables such as broccoli, cauliflower, and kale. These foods contain compounds that help to support healthy hormone balance.

Maintaining Meridian Balance for Optimal Health

Meridians are pathways through which energy flows in the human body. There are twelve major meridians that correspond to different organs and body functions. Keeping these meridians in balance is important for optimal health. Meridian imbalances can lead to various physical and emotional problems. Below we will discuss how to maintain meridian balance for optimal health.

One way to maintain meridian balance is through regular exercise. Physical activities such as yoga, tai chi, and qigong can help to balance the flow of energy in the body. These exercises involve gentle movements that stretch and strengthen the body while also promoting relaxation and mental clarity. Yoga, for example, has specific poses that target different meridians, such as the lung and heart meridians, which help to stimulate energy flow and promote healing.

Another way to maintain meridian balance is through acupuncture. Acupuncture is a traditional Chinese medicine technique that involves inserting thin needles into specific points on the body to balance the flow of energy. By stimulating the acupuncture points along the meridians, acupuncture helps to improve the flow of energy and promote healing. It can also help to alleviate pain and reduce stress.

In addition to acupuncture, acupressure is another technique that can be used to balance the meridians. Acupressure involves applying pressure to specific points on the body, which helps to stimulate the flow of energy and promote healing. This can be done using the fingers, thumbs, or special acupressure tools.

Nutrition also plays a critical role in maintaining meridian balance. Eating a healthy and balanced diet that is rich in whole foods can help to support the functioning of the organs and body systems that correspond to the different meridians. For example, the liver meridian is associated with detoxification and digestion, so eating foods that support these functions, such as leafy greens, cruciferous vegetables, and bitter foods, can help to keep this meridian in balance.

Another important aspect of maintaining meridian balance is to manage stress. Stress can disrupt the flow of energy in the body and lead to imbalances. Practices such as meditation, deep breathing, and mindfulness can help to reduce stress and promote relaxation, which in turn helps to balance the meridians.

It is also important to pay attention to the quality of the air we breathe and the water we drink. Pollution and toxins in the environment can negatively affect the flow of energy in the body and disrupt the functioning of the organs and body systems that correspond to the meridians. Drinking clean water and avoiding exposure to environmental toxins can help to support meridian health.

Another way to maintain meridian balance is to get enough restful sleep. Sleep is a critical time for the body to repair and restore itself. Lack of sleep can disrupt the flow of energy in the body and lead to meridian imbalances. Getting at least 7-8 hours of sleep per night can help to promote meridian balance and support overall health.

Finally, it is important to seek out professional help if there are persistent issues with meridian balance. A licensed acupuncturist or other traditional Chinese medicine practitioner can assess meridian imbalances and recommend appropriate treatments, such as acupuncture, acupressure, herbal remedies, or dietary and lifestyle changes.

The Importance of Regular Meridian Care

The concept of meridians is central to traditional Chinese medicine (TCM) and involves a network of channels in the body that transport energy, known as qi or chi. These meridians are believed to influence the functioning of different organs and systems in the body, as well as overall health and well-being. While there are twelve major meridians, it is important to maintain balance in all of them for optimal health.

Meridian care involves a variety of practices, including acupuncture, acupressure, moxibustion, cupping therapy, qigong, and meditation, among others. Regular care of the meridians is essential to maintain balance and prevent blockages that can result in illness and disease.

One of the main reasons for the importance of regular meridian care is that the meridians can become blocked, preventing the free flow of qi throughout the body. Blockages can occur due to stress, poor diet, lack of exercise, or physical injury, among other factors. When the flow of qi is blocked, it can lead to a variety of physical and emotional symptoms, including pain, fatigue, anxiety, and depression.

Acupuncture and acupressure are two common practices used to unblock the meridians and restore balance to the body. Acupuncture involves the use of thin needles inserted into specific points along the meridians, while acupressure involves applying pressure to these same points using the fingers or other tools. Both practices stimulate the flow of qi and promote healing throughout the body.

Moxibustion is another practice used in meridian care that involves the burning of dried mugwort to stimulate the flow of qi and promote healing. Cupping therapy involves the use of suction cups placed on specific points along the meridians to promote blood flow and alleviate pain and tension.

Qigong and meditation are practices used to balance the mind, body, and spirit, and promote overall health and well-being. Qigong involves gentle movements, breathing exercises, and meditation techniques designed to balance the flow of qi throughout the body. Meditation involves a variety of techniques designed to quiet the mind and promote relaxation, which can also help to restore balance to the meridians.

In addition to these practices, nutrition also plays a crucial role in meridian care. Foods that support meridian health include fresh fruits and vegetables, whole grains, lean protein sources, and healthy fats. Foods to avoid include processed foods, sugar, caffeine, and alcohol, which can disrupt the flow of qi and lead to blockages.

Maintaining regular meridian care is essential to support overall health and well-being. Practices such as acupuncture, acupressure, moxibustion, cupping therapy, qigong, and meditation can all be incorporated into a regular self-care routine to promote balance and prevent illness and disease. In addition, eating a balanced diet that supports meridian health can further enhance the benefits of these practices.

Lifestyle Tips for Supporting Meridian Health

The concept of meridians in traditional Chinese medicine (TCM) describes a network of energy channels that flow throughout the body, connecting different organs and tissues. These meridians are essential to the practice of acupuncture, acupressure, and other TCM therapies. While meridian health is primarily addressed through these therapies, there are also lifestyle tips that can support overall meridian balance and health.

Exercise regularly: Regular physical activity can help promote blood and energy flow throughout the body, which is essential for meridian health. Practices such as tai chi and qigong are especially beneficial as they focus on gentle movements that promote the flow of energy throughout the body.

Maintain a balanced diet: A balanced diet that includes a variety of fresh fruits, vegetables, whole grains, and lean protein can help ensure that the body receives the nutrients it needs to function properly. In TCM, foods are also categorized according to their energetic properties, so it's important to eat foods that are appropriate for your individual constitution and health needs.

Stay hydrated: Water is essential for maintaining proper bodily functions and promoting the flow of energy throughout the body. It's important to drink enough water each day to ensure that the body stays hydrated.

Practice stress management: Stress can cause imbalances in the body's energy flow, which can lead to meridian blockages and other health issues. Practices such as meditation, deep breathing exercises, and yoga can help reduce stress and promote meridian balance.

Get enough rest: Adequate sleep is essential for maintaining overall health and promoting proper energy flow throughout the body. It's important to get enough rest each night to ensure that the body has time to repair and rejuvenate.

Avoid toxins: Exposure to toxins such as cigarette smoke, pollution, and certain chemicals can disrupt the body's energy flow and lead to meridian blockages. It's important to avoid exposure to these toxins as much as possible and to take steps to support the body's natural detoxification processes.

Practice self-care: Taking time for self-care activities such as getting a massage, taking a relaxing bath, or practicing aromatherapy can help promote relaxation and support overall meridian health.

Seek regular meridian therapy: Regular acupuncture, acupressure, or other meridian-based therapies can help promote energy flow throughout the body, reduce meridian blockages, and support overall health and well-being.

Emotional and Mental Health and the Meridians

Emotional and mental health is an essential aspect of overall well-being, and it is closely related to the meridian system in traditional Chinese medicine (TCM). In TCM, it is believed that the mind and emotions are intimately linked with the physical body, and that imbalances in one can lead to imbalances in the other. The meridian system plays a crucial role in this relationship, as it is responsible for the flow of qi (life force energy) throughout the body, including the organs and tissues associated with emotional and mental health.

According to TCM theory, each meridian is associated with an organ system and an element. The organs associated with emotional and mental health are the heart, spleen, liver, lungs, and kidneys. Each organ system is also associated with certain emotions, and imbalances in these emotions can lead to blockages in the corresponding meridians.

The heart meridian is associated with joy, and imbalances can manifest as restlessness, anxiety, and insomnia. The spleen meridian is associated with worry, and imbalances can manifest as obsessive thoughts, poor concentration, and overthinking. The liver meridian is associated with anger, and imbalances can manifest as irritability, frustration, and depression. The lungs meridian is associated with grief, and imbalances can manifest as sadness, melancholy, and feeling stuck. The kidneys meridian is associated with fear, and imbalances can manifest as phobias, anxiety, and panic attacks.

There are several meridian-based techniques that can help support emotional and mental health. Acupuncture, acupressure, and moxibustion can all be used to stimulate the flow of qi and help to balance the meridians. Acupuncture involves the insertion of thin needles into specific points along the meridians, while acupressure involves applying pressure to these points with the fingers or hands. Moxibustion involves burning dried mugwort over the meridian points to warm and stimulate them.

In addition to these techniques, lifestyle factors such as diet, exercise, and stress management can also play a role in supporting emotional and mental health. Eating a balanced diet rich in whole foods, practicing regular physical activity, and engaging in relaxation techniques such as meditation or yoga can all help to support the flow of qi and balance the meridians.

It is important to note that emotional and mental health concerns should always be addressed by a qualified healthcare professional. While meridian-based techniques can be helpful in supporting emotional and mental health, they should be used in conjunction with other treatments such as therapy or medication, as appropriate.

The Connection Between Emotions and Meridian Health

The meridian system is a complex network of energy pathways that flows through the body, according to Traditional Chinese Medicine (TCM). Each meridian is associated with a specific organ or organ system, as well as a particular emotion or set of emotions. In TCM, the relationship between emotions and meridian health is considered to be a key factor in achieving overall wellness.

According to TCM, emotions are seen as a normal and natural part of life, and it is when emotions are repressed or not expressed in a healthy way that they can become problematic. Each meridian is thought to be associated with a particular emotion or set of emotions, and when that emotion is not expressed or is expressed in an unhealthy way, it can lead to an imbalance in the corresponding meridian.

For example, the liver meridian is associated with the emotion of anger, and when anger is not expressed in a healthy way, it can lead to liver meridian imbalances such as headaches, eye problems, and menstrual irregularities. The lung meridian is associated with the emotion of grief, and when grief is not expressed in a healthy way, it can lead to lung meridian imbalances such as respiratory issues, skin problems, and immune system deficiencies.

In TCM, it is believed that meridian imbalances can also lead to emotional imbalances, creating a feedback loop that can be difficult to break. For example, if a person is experiencing a liver meridian imbalance due to repressed anger, it can lead to further feelings of frustration, irritability, and anger, perpetuating the imbalance.

In addition to the connection between emotions and meridian health, TCM also recognizes the impact of stress on the body and the meridian system. Chronic stress can lead to meridian imbalances, particularly in the kidney and adrenal meridians, which are associated with the body's stress response.

To support emotional and mental health through the meridian system, TCM offers a variety of approaches, including acupuncture, acupressure, herbal medicine, and dietary therapy. Acupuncture and acupressure can help to rebalance the meridians by stimulating the flow of energy through the body and releasing any blockages or stagnation.

Herbal medicine can also be used to support emotional and mental health, with different herbs being chosen based on the specific meridian imbalances present. For example, the herb Rhodiola is commonly used to support the adrenal meridian and reduce stress, while the herb Reishi is used to support the lung meridian and promote feelings of calm and relaxation.

Dietary therapy is also an important aspect of supporting emotional and mental health through the meridian system. In TCM, different foods are believed to have different energetic properties, and choosing foods that support the specific meridian imbalances present can help to rebalance the meridian system and support overall wellness. For example, foods that are bitter in taste, such as dark leafy greens and bitter melon, are believed to support the liver meridian and promote healthy emotional expression.

In addition to these traditional approaches, there are also lifestyle factors that can support emotional and mental health through the meridian system. Regular exercise, adequate sleep, and stress-reduction techniques such as meditation and yoga can all help to support a healthy and balanced meridian system.

Techniques for Balancing Emotions Through Meridian Work

The human body is a complex system, and the meridian system plays a significant role in regulating its functions. Meridians are channels that run throughout the body and are responsible for the flow of energy or Qi. In Traditional Chinese Medicine, it is believed that emotions affect the meridians, and an imbalance in one can lead to an imbalance in the other. Therefore, to maintain optimal health, it is essential to maintain balance in both physical and emotional aspects. Below we will discuss techniques for balancing emotions through meridian work.

Meridian Work

Meridian work is a holistic approach that combines various techniques to restore balance to the body. The following techniques can be used to balance emotions through meridian work:

Acupuncture: Acupuncture is an ancient Chinese practice that involves inserting needles into specific points on the body to stimulate the flow of Qi. Acupuncture is believed to balance emotions by stimulating the meridians and regulating the flow of energy. It is a safe and effective method that can be used to treat various emotional imbalances such as anxiety, depression, and stress.

Acupressure: Acupressure is a technique that involves applying pressure to specific points on the body. The pressure is applied with the fingers, hands, or elbows to stimulate the flow of Qi. Acupressure is believed to balance emotions by unblocking the meridians, thus allowing the energy to flow freely. It is a non-invasive technique that can be done at home or with the help of a practitioner.

Moxibustion: Moxibustion is a technique that involves burning the herb mugwort near specific acupuncture points to stimulate the flow of Qi. Moxibustion is believed to balance emotions by warming and invigorating the meridians. It is a gentle and effective method that can be used to treat emotional imbalances such as anxiety, depression, and stress.

Cupping: Cupping is a technique that involves placing cups on the skin and creating a vacuum. The vacuum is created either by heat or suction. Cupping is believed to balance emotions by unblocking the meridians, thus allowing the energy to flow freely. It is a non-invasive technique that can be done at home or with the help of a practitioner.

Emotional Balancing Techniques

In addition to meridian work, the following techniques can also be used to balance emotions:

Meditation: Meditation is a technique that involves focusing the mind on a particular object or thought. Meditation is believed to balance emotions by calming the mind and reducing stress. It is a powerful tool that can be used to treat various emotional imbalances such as anxiety, depression, and stress.

Breathing Exercises: Breathing exercises are a technique that involves controlling the breath to calm the mind and reduce stress. Breathing exercises are believed to balance emotions by calming the mind and reducing stress. They are a simple and effective technique that can be done at home or anywhere.

Yoga: Yoga is a physical practice that involves various postures and breathing exercises. Yoga is believed to balance emotions by improving the flow of energy in the body and reducing stress. It is a gentle and effective method that can be used to treat emotional imbalances such as anxiety, depression, and stress.

Herbal Remedies: Herbal remedies are a natural and safe way to balance emotions. Certain herbs such as chamomile, lavender, and passionflower are known to have a calming effect on the mind and can be used to treat various emotional imbalances such as anxiety, depression, and stress.

Meridian Massage Techniques

Meridian massage is a form of bodywork that focuses on the 12 major meridians in the body. These meridians are pathways through which energy or Qi flows, and they are closely linked to various bodily functions and emotions. The goal of meridian massage is to balance the flow of Qi in these meridians, which can lead to improved health and wellbeing.

Meridian massage techniques can vary depending on the practitioner and the goals of the session. However, there are some common techniques that are used in many meridian massage sessions.

One common technique is acupressure, which involves applying pressure to specific points along the meridians. These points are called acupoints, and they are believed to be areas where Qi is more easily accessible. By applying pressure to these points, the practitioner can help to release blockages and restore the flow of Qi.

Another technique used in meridian massage is tapping, also known as percussion. This involves using the fingertips or a small instrument to tap along the meridians. Tapping is thought to stimulate the flow of Qi and help to break up blockages.

Meridian massage may also involve stretching or gentle movement along the meridians. This can help to improve flexibility and release tension in the muscles and connective tissues surrounding the meridians.

In addition to these techniques, some practitioners may incorporate other forms of bodywork, such as Swedish massage or deep tissue massage, into their meridian massage sessions. These techniques can help to relax the body and promote a sense of wellbeing.

The benefits of meridian massage are many. By balancing the flow of Qi in the meridians, this form of bodywork can help to improve a wide range of health issues. For example, meridian massage may be beneficial for those experiencing digestive issues, headaches, menstrual cramps, and chronic pain. It may also help to reduce stress and anxiety, improve sleep quality, and boost the immune system.

In addition to its physical benefits, meridian massage can also have emotional and psychological benefits. The meridians are closely linked to different emotions, and imbalances in the flow of Qi can lead to emotional and mental health issues. By restoring balance to the meridians, meridian massage can help to reduce feelings of anxiety, depression, and anger, and promote a sense of calm and relaxation.

It is important to note that meridian massage should be performed by a trained and licensed practitioner. While this form of bodywork is generally safe, it may not be appropriate for those with certain health conditions, such as cancer or blood disorders. It is always best to consult with a healthcare provider before trying any new form of bodywork.

Introduction to Meridian Massage

Meridian massage is a traditional Chinese medicine practice that focuses on the energy channels, known as meridians, that run through the body. In this massage technique, pressure is applied to specific points along the meridians to help balance the flow of energy and promote overall health and wellbeing.

The concept of meridian massage is based on the idea that energy, or Qi (pronounced "chee"), flows through the body along specific pathways, or meridians. This energy is said to nourish and support the various organs, tissues, and systems of the body, and an imbalance in this energy can lead to a variety of health problems.

Meridian massage aims to address these imbalances by applying pressure to specific points along the meridians, known as acupressure points. By applying pressure to these points, the flow of energy is stimulated, helping to restore balance and promote healing.

There are 12 major meridians in the body, each of which is associated with a different organ or system. These include the lung, large intestine, stomach, spleen, heart, small intestine, bladder, kidney, pericardium, triple warmer, gallbladder, and liver meridians.

Each meridian has a specific pathway through the body and is associated with certain acupressure points. For example, the lung meridian runs from the chest to the thumb and is associated with points along this pathway, while the kidney meridian runs from the sole of the foot to the chest and has corresponding points along this pathway.

Meridian massage typically involves using fingers, thumbs, or other tools to apply pressure to these acupressure points along the meridians. The pressure can be gentle or firm, depending on the individual's needs and preferences.

In addition to promoting energy balance, meridian massage is also thought to have a number of other health benefits. For example, it may help to reduce stress and anxiety, relieve pain and tension, improve circulation, and boost the immune system.

There are many different techniques and styles of meridian massage, each with its own unique approach and focus. Some therapists may incorporate other modalities, such as aromatherapy or reflexology, into their meridian massage sessions to further enhance the therapeutic benefits.

How to Perform a Meridian Massage

Meridian massage is a powerful therapy that aims to balance the energy flow in the body's meridian system. It is an ancient healing technique that has been used for centuries to relieve pain, tension, and stress. The concept behind meridian massage is that each meridian point in the body is linked to an organ and that applying pressure to these points can help to unblock energy flow and restore balance to the body.

Before performing a meridian massage, it's important to understand the basic principles of the meridian system. The meridian system is made up of 12 main channels or pathways that connect different organs in the body. These channels are divided into six yin and six yang meridians, and each is associated with one of the five elements: wood, fire, earth, metal, and water.

To perform a meridian massage, you will need to identify the meridian points that correspond to the specific ailment you wish to treat. This can be done by consulting with a trained practitioner or by using a meridian chart or map. Once you have identified the meridian points, you can begin to apply pressure to them using your fingers, thumbs, palms, or knuckles.

It's important to apply pressure to the meridian points gradually and gently, using a circular or rubbing motion. The pressure should be firm enough to stimulate the point but not so strong as to cause discomfort or pain. As you apply pressure, it's important to focus on your breathing and to stay relaxed.

To enhance the effects of the massage, you can also use essential oils or herbal ointments. These can be applied to the meridian points before or during the massage to help stimulate the energy flow and enhance the therapeutic effects of the massage.

There are many different techniques and styles of meridian massage, each with its own unique approach and focus. Some of the most common techniques include acupressure, shiatsu, and reflexology.

Acupressure involves applying pressure to specific meridian points using the fingers, palms, or elbows. This technique is often used to relieve tension and pain in the body, and it can also help to improve circulation and promote relaxation.

Shiatsu is a form of Japanese massage that involves applying pressure to the meridian points using the fingers, palms, or elbows. It is often used to relieve tension and pain in the muscles and joints, and it can also help to improve circulation and promote relaxation.

Reflexology is a type of massage that focuses on the feet, hands, and ears. It involves applying pressure to specific reflex points that correspond to different organs and systems in the body. Reflexology is often used to promote relaxation, improve circulation, and relieve pain and tension in the body.

Essential Oils and the Meridians

Essential oils have been used for centuries for their therapeutic properties, and their use has become increasingly popular in recent years. When used in conjunction with meridian therapy, essential oils can help to balance and harmonize the flow of energy in the body. Below we will explore the relationship between essential oils and the meridians, and how this can promote optimal health.

The meridian system is the basis of traditional Chinese medicine and acupuncture. It is a complex network of energy pathways that run throughout the body, connecting the major organs, tissues, and systems. There are 12 major meridians, each of which corresponds to a specific organ or function in the body. These meridians are said to be responsible for the flow of energy or "qi" through the body. When this flow is disrupted, it can lead to physical, emotional, and mental imbalances.

Essential oils are highly concentrated plant extracts that are known for their therapeutic properties. They are extracted from various parts of plants, including leaves, flowers, bark, and roots. Each essential oil has a unique chemical composition that gives it specific therapeutic properties. For example, lavender essential oil is known for its calming and relaxing properties, while peppermint essential oil is energizing and invigorating.

When essential oils are applied to the skin, they are absorbed into the bloodstream and can have a powerful effect on the body. When used in conjunction with meridian therapy, essential oils can help to balance the flow of energy through the meridians, promoting optimal health and wellbeing.

There are several ways to use essential oils for meridian therapy. One of the most effective methods is to apply them directly to the skin along the meridian lines. This can be done by diluting the essential oil with a carrier oil, such as coconut oil or almond oil, and applying it to the skin in a gentle, circular motion.

Another method is to inhale the essential oils using a diffuser or by placing a few drops on a tissue or handkerchief. This can be particularly effective for balancing the energy in the lungs and respiratory system, which are connected to the lung meridian.

Certain essential oils are particularly beneficial for specific meridians. For example, peppermint essential oil is said to be particularly effective for the stomach meridian, while lavender essential oil is beneficial for the heart meridian. By using the appropriate essential oil for each meridian, it is possible to achieve a more targeted and effective treatment.

In addition to their therapeutic properties, essential oils can also have a powerful emotional impact. Many essential oils are known for their ability to promote relaxation, reduce anxiety, and lift the mood. By incorporating essential oils into meridian therapy, it is possible to address both the physical and emotional aspects of health and wellbeing.

It is important to note that essential oils should be used with caution and under the guidance of a qualified practitioner. Some essential oils can be irritating to the skin or may cause allergic reactions in some individuals. It is also important to ensure that the essential oils are of high quality and pure, as adulterated oils may not have the same therapeutic properties.

Introduction to Essential Oils

Essential oils have been used for centuries for their therapeutic properties, and are commonly used in aromatherapy for promoting relaxation, reducing stress and anxiety, and improving overall well-being. Essential oils are extracted from various parts of plants, including leaves, flowers, roots, and bark, and are highly concentrated natural plant extracts that contain volatile aromatic compounds.

The use of essential oils in traditional Chinese medicine is also well documented. In TCM, essential oils are used to balance the energy flow in the body by working with the meridian system. The meridian system is a network of channels that run throughout the body, and through which Qi, the vital energy of the body, flows. By using essential oils to stimulate specific meridians, TCM practitioners can help to restore balance and promote healing.

One of the most important aspects of essential oils in TCM is their ability to work with the Five Elements, which are Wood, Fire, Earth, Metal, and Water. Each element corresponds to specific organs, emotions, and meridians in the body, and essential oils can be used to support the health and balance of each element.

Essential oils can be used in several ways to support meridian health. One of the most common methods is through inhalation. When essential oils are inhaled, they stimulate the olfactory system, which is linked to the limbic system in the brain, where emotions and memories are processed. The limbic system is also connected to the autonomic nervous system, which regulates bodily functions such as heart rate, breathing, and digestion. By inhaling essential oils, we can stimulate specific meridians and support the flow of Qi in the body.

Another way to use essential oils for meridian health is through topical application. Essential oils can be diluted in carrier oils such as jojoba or coconut oil, and applied directly to the skin over specific meridians. This method allows the oils to be absorbed into the bloodstream, where they can support overall meridian health and balance.

When using essential oils in TCM, it is important to choose oils that are appropriate for the specific meridian being treated. For example, if working with the Lung meridian, oils such as eucalyptus, peppermint, and lavender may be used to support respiratory health and promote relaxation. When working with the Liver meridian, oils such as rosemary, ginger, and grapefruit may be used to promote detoxification and support healthy digestion.

In addition to their therapeutic benefits, essential oils also offer a natural alternative to conventional medicines, which can have negative side effects. Essential oils are generally safe when used properly, but it is important to work with a trained TCM practitioner to ensure that they are being used correctly and safely.

Using Essential Oils for Meridian Health

Essential oils have been used for thousands of years in traditional healing practices for their medicinal properties. They are extracted from various parts of plants and are known to have a wide range of therapeutic effects on the body, mind, and spirit. In Traditional Chinese Medicine (TCM), essential oils are often used to support the health of the meridian system, which is considered to be the body's energy pathways.

The meridian system is the foundation of TCM, and it is believed that every organ and function of the body is connected to a specific meridian. These meridians are channels that run throughout the body, carrying energy, or Qi, to all parts of the body. When there is an imbalance in the flow of Qi through the meridians, it can lead to physical, emotional, and mental health problems. Essential oils can help to restore balance to the meridian system and support overall health and well-being.

One of the primary ways that essential oils are used for meridian health is through aromatherapy. Aromatherapy is the practice of using essential oils for therapeutic purposes by inhaling their aromas. When inhaled, the molecules of the essential oils enter the body through the nasal cavity and are carried through the bloodstream to different parts of the body, including the meridians. Different essential oils have different effects on the body and can be used to support specific meridians and organs.

For example, peppermint oil is known to stimulate the liver and gallbladder meridians, while lavender oil is used to calm the heart and balance the lung meridian. Eucalyptus oil is commonly used to support the respiratory system and open the lung meridian, while ginger oil can be used to warm the stomach and spleen meridians.

Essential oils can also be used topically to support meridian health. This is done by diluting the essential oil in a carrier oil, such as jojoba or almond oil, and applying it to specific points along the meridians. This technique is similar to acupuncture, but instead of needles, essential oils are used to stimulate the meridians.

There are twelve primary meridians in the body, and each one is associated with specific organs and functions. For example, the lung meridian is associated with the lungs, skin, and immune system, while the liver meridian is associated with the liver, gallbladder, and eyes. By applying essential oils to specific points along these meridians, it is possible to support the health of the associated organs and functions.

In addition to supporting physical health, essential oils can also have a profound effect on emotional and mental health. Many essential oils have a calming effect on the nervous system and can be used to reduce stress and anxiety. For example, lavender oil is known for its calming and relaxing properties, while bergamot oil is often used to uplift the mood and reduce feelings of depression.

When using essential oils for meridian health, it is important to use high-quality, pure essential oils. Synthetic oils or oils that have been adulterated with other substances may not have the same therapeutic effects and could even be harmful to the body. It is also important to dilute the essential oils in a carrier oil before applying them topically to avoid skin irritation.

The Connection Between Meridians and Chakras

The concept of meridians has been widely studied and utilized in traditional Chinese medicine for centuries. However, in recent years, the connection between meridians and chakras has become a topic of interest for those interested in holistic health and well-being. Below we will explore the relationship between meridians and chakras and how they can work together to promote optimal health.

Meridians are the pathways in the body through which vital energy, or qi, flows. According to traditional Chinese medicine, there are twelve major meridians, each corresponding to an organ system in the body. These meridians are connected to specific acupressure points that can be stimulated to promote balance and harmony in the body. By working with the meridians, practitioners of traditional Chinese medicine can identify imbalances and blockages in the body's energy flow and use various techniques to restore balance.

Chakras, on the other hand, are energy centers in the body that are believed to correspond to different aspects of our physical, emotional, and spiritual health. There are seven major chakras, each located along the spine, from the base of the spine to the top of the head. Each chakra is associated with a specific color, element, and sound, and is thought to govern different aspects of our physical, emotional, and spiritual health.

While meridians and chakras are different concepts, they are closely related. The meridians are considered to be the physical manifestation of the body's energy flow, while the chakras are the energetic centers that regulate that flow. In other words, the meridians are the pathways through which energy flows, while the chakras are the centers of that energy.

There are several ways in which practitioners can work with both the meridians and chakras to promote health and well-being. One approach is to use acupressure and acupuncture techniques to stimulate the meridians and restore balance to the body's energy flow. By working with specific acupressure points, practitioners can target imbalances and blockages in the meridians, promoting optimal flow and restoring balance to the body.

Another approach is to use meditation and visualization techniques to balance the chakras. By focusing on each chakra and its associated color, element, and sound, practitioners can bring awareness and balance to each energy center. This can help to release any blockages or imbalances in the chakras, allowing energy to flow freely throughout the body.

In addition to acupressure, acupuncture, and meditation, there are other approaches that can be used to promote the balance of both meridians and chakras. These include yoga, tai chi, qigong, and other forms of movement and exercise that are designed to promote the flow of energy throughout the body.

In order to work with both meridians and chakras effectively, it is important to have a basic understanding of both systems. This can be accomplished through research, study, and working with a qualified practitioner. By working with these systems together, it is possible to promote optimal health and well-being, both physically and energetically.

The Chakra System Explained

The chakra system is an ancient Indian system of energy centers in the body that are said to regulate physical, mental, and emotional well-being. The word "chakra" means "wheel" in Sanskrit, and each chakra is thought to be like a spinning wheel of energy.

There are seven main chakras in the body, each associated with a specific color, location, and set of functions. The first chakra, called the root chakra, is located at the base of the spine and is associated with the color red. It is said to govern issues of physical survival, such as food, shelter, and safety.

The second chakra, known as the sacral chakra, is located in the lower abdomen and is associated with the color orange. It is said to govern creativity, sexuality, and emotional well-being.

The third chakra, called the solar plexus chakra, is located in the upper abdomen and is associated with the color yellow. It is said to govern personal power, self-esteem, and the ability to take action.

The fourth chakra, known as the heart chakra, is located in the center of the chest and is associated with the color green. It is said to govern love, compassion, and emotional balance.

The fifth chakra, called the throat chakra, is located in the throat and is associated with the color blue. It is said to govern communication, self-expression, and creativity.

The sixth chakra, known as the third eye chakra, is located in the forehead and is associated with the color indigo. It is said to govern intuition, spiritual awareness, and the ability to see beyond the physical realm.

The seventh chakra, called the crown chakra, is located at the top of the head and is associated with the color violet. It is said to govern connection to the divine, spiritual enlightenment, and transcendence.

The chakra system is closely related to the meridian system of Traditional Chinese Medicine, as both systems involve the flow of energy throughout the body. In Chinese medicine, the meridians are thought to be pathways through which Qi, or life force energy, flows. Each meridian is associated with a specific organ or bodily function.

While the chakra system is not recognized by Western medicine, many people believe that balancing the chakras can help to promote physical, mental, and emotional health. There are a variety of techniques that can be used to balance the chakras, including meditation, yoga, visualization, and energy healing practices such as Reiki.

In addition to balancing the chakras, it is also important to maintain healthy meridian flow in order to promote overall health and well-being. This can be achieved through a variety of practices, including acupuncture, acupressure, meridian massage, and energy work.

Ultimately, the chakra and meridian systems provide a holistic approach to health and wellness, acknowledging the interconnectedness of the physical, emotional, and spiritual aspects of our being. By working with these systems, we can cultivate greater balance, harmony, and vitality in our lives.

The Relationship Between Meridians and Chakras

The concept of energy flow through the body is central to both traditional Chinese medicine and Indian Ayurveda. In Chinese medicine, this energy is called "Qi" (pronounced "chee"), and it is believed to flow through channels in the body called "meridians". In Ayurveda, the energy is called "prana", and it flows through channels called "nadis". While there are some differences in terminology and approach, both systems share the belief that this energy flow is vital to health and well-being.

In addition to meridians, Chinese medicine also recognizes a system of energy centers called "acupuncture points". These points are believed to correspond to specific organs and functions in the body. In Ayurveda, the energy centers are known as "chakras". There are seven major chakras in the body, each of which is believed to correspond to a different aspect of the self, including physical, emotional, and spiritual health.

The concept of chakras can be traced back to ancient India, where they were first mentioned in the Vedas, a collection of sacred texts dating back to 1500 BCE. According to Ayurvedic tradition, the chakras are spinning wheels of energy that run along the spine, with each chakra corresponding to a different part of the body and a different aspect of the self.

The seven major chakras are as follows:

Root Chakra (Muladhara): Located at the base of the spine, this chakra is associated with survival and groundedness. It is connected to the earth element and is related to the adrenal glands and the immune system.

Sacral Chakra (Svadhisthana): Located in the lower abdomen, this chakra is associated with pleasure and creativity. It is connected to the water element and is related to the reproductive system and the kidneys.

Solar Plexus Chakra (Manipura): Located in the upper abdomen, this chakra is associated with personal power and self-confidence. It is connected to the fire element and is related to the digestive system and the liver.

Heart Chakra (Anahata): Located in the center of the chest, this chakra is associated with love and compassion. It is connected to the air element and is related to the circulatory system and the heart.

Throat Chakra (Vishuddha): Located in the throat, this chakra is associated with communication and self-expression. It is connected to the ether element and is related to the respiratory system and the thyroid gland.

Third Eye Chakra (Ajna): Located in the center of the forehead, this chakra is associated with intuition and inner wisdom. It is connected to the light element and is related to the nervous system and the pituitary gland.

Crown Chakra (Sahasrara): Located at the top of the head, this chakra is associated with spiritual enlightenment and unity. It is connected to the space element and is related to the pineal gland and the central nervous system.

While chakras and meridians are different systems, there is a growing body of evidence to suggest that they are closely related. For example, many of the acupuncture points correspond to specific chakras in the body. In addition, both systems are based on the idea that energy flow through the body is essential for good health, and both emphasize the importance of balance and harmony in this energy flow.

Common Meridian Imbalances and Their Symptoms

The meridian system is an important aspect of traditional Chinese medicine, and it is believed to play a vital role in the overall health of the body. The meridians are pathways through which energy, or qi, flows through the body. Each meridian is associated with a specific organ system and is responsible for the proper functioning of that system. When a meridian is blocked or imbalanced, it can result in a variety of physical and emotional symptoms. Below we will explore common meridian imbalances and their symptoms.

Lung Meridian Imbalances: The lung meridian is associated with the respiratory system and is responsible for the proper functioning of the lungs. Imbalances in this meridian can result in respiratory issues such as coughing, wheezing, and shortness of breath. Emotional imbalances associated with the lung meridian include sadness, grief, and depression.

Large Intestine Meridian Imbalances: The large intestine meridian is associated with the digestive system and is responsible for the proper functioning of the large intestine. Imbalances in this meridian can result in digestive issues such as constipation, diarrhea, and abdominal pain. Emotional imbalances associated with the large intestine meridian include difficulty letting go of emotions and feelings of sadness.

Stomach Meridian Imbalances: The stomach meridian is associated with the digestive system and is responsible for the proper functioning of the stomach. Imbalances in this meridian can result in digestive issues such as nausea, vomiting, and acid reflux. Emotional imbalances associated with the stomach meridian include worry, anxiety, and overthinking.

Spleen Meridian Imbalances: The spleen meridian is associated with the digestive system and is responsible for the proper functioning of the spleen. Imbalances in this meridian can result in digestive issues such as bloating, gas, and poor digestion. Emotional imbalances associated with the spleen meridian include worry, overthinking, and a lack of grounding.

Heart Meridian Imbalances: The heart meridian is associated with the cardiovascular system and is responsible for the proper functioning of the heart. Imbalances in this meridian can result in cardiovascular issues such as palpitations, arrhythmias, and high blood pressure. Emotional imbalances associated with the heart meridian include anxiety, nervousness, and lack of joy.

Small Intestine Meridian Imbalances: The small intestine meridian is associated with the digestive system and is responsible for the proper functioning of the small intestine. Imbalances in this meridian can result in digestive issues such as bloating, gas, and abdominal pain. Emotional imbalances associated with the small intestine meridian include difficulty making decisions and lack of clarity.

Bladder Meridian Imbalances: The bladder meridian is associated with the urinary system and is responsible for the proper functioning of the bladder. Imbalances in this meridian can result in urinary issues such as frequent urination, painful urination, and urinary tract infections. Emotional imbalances associated with the bladder meridian include fear, anxiety, and lack of trust.

Kidney Meridian Imbalances: The kidney meridian is associated with the urinary system and is responsible for the proper functioning of the kidneys. Imbalances in this meridian can result in urinary issues such as frequent urination, painful urination, and urinary tract infections. Emotional imbalances associated with the kidney meridian include fear, anxiety, and lack of trust.

Pericardium Meridian Imbalances: The pericardium meridian is associated with the cardiovascular system and is responsible for the proper functioning of the pericardium. Imbalances in this meridian can result in cardiovascular issues such as palpitations, arrhythmias, and high blood pressure.

Recognizing Meridian Imbalances

The meridian system is a complex network of energy channels in the body that are responsible for the flow of vital life force energy, or Qi. When this flow is disrupted or blocked, it can result in a wide range of physical, emotional, and mental imbalances. In order to maintain optimal health, it is important to be able to recognize the signs and symptoms of meridian imbalances.

There are twelve major meridians in the body, each of which is associated with a particular organ or organ system. By understanding the function of each meridian and the signs and symptoms of imbalances, it is possible to identify areas of the body that may need extra attention and care.

One common meridian imbalance is known as Qi deficiency. This occurs when there is a lack of energy flowing through the meridian, resulting in fatigue, weakness, and lethargy. Symptoms may also include pale skin, shortness of breath, and a weak pulse. Qi deficiency is often associated with the Spleen and Stomach meridians, which are responsible for digestion and nutrient absorption.

Another common meridian imbalance is known as Qi stagnation. This occurs when energy becomes blocked or stagnant in a particular meridian, resulting in pain, tension, and discomfort. Symptoms may include headaches, menstrual cramps, and digestive issues. Qi stagnation is often associated with the Liver and Gallbladder meridians, which are responsible for the smooth flow of energy throughout the body.

A third common meridian imbalance is known as Yin deficiency. This occurs when there is a lack of nourishing Yin energy in the body, resulting in symptoms such as dry skin, hot flashes, and insomnia. Yin deficiency is often associated with the Kidney and Heart meridians, which are responsible for regulating body fluids and maintaining emotional balance.

In addition to these specific imbalances, there are also a number of general signs and symptoms that may indicate meridian imbalances. These can include chronic pain, mood swings, fatigue, and digestive issues. It is important to pay attention to these symptoms and seek out the appropriate meridian-based therapies to address any imbalances.

There are a variety of techniques and therapies that can be used to correct meridian imbalances. These can include acupuncture, acupressure, massage, herbal remedies, and dietary changes. The goal of these therapies is to restore the flow of Qi through the affected meridian, allowing the body to heal and rebalance itself naturally.

Acupuncture, for example, involves the insertion of tiny needles into specific acupoints along the meridian. This stimulates the flow of Qi, helping to restore balance and alleviate symptoms. Acupressure, on the other hand, involves applying pressure to specific acupoints with the fingers or hands. This can be done at home or with the help of a trained practitioner.

Massage is another effective way to address meridian imbalances. By applying pressure to specific areas of the body, a massage therapist can help to stimulate the flow of Qi and promote healing. Herbal remedies can also be used to address meridian imbalances, with many traditional Chinese herbs having specific actions on particular meridians.

Finally, dietary changes can be an effective way to address meridian imbalances. Certain foods are believed to have specific effects on the meridians and can be used to support healing and balance. For example, foods that are sour are believed to stimulate the Liver meridian, while foods that are sweet are believed to support the Spleen meridian.

Addressing Imbalances Through Meridian Work

Meridian work is a holistic approach that aims to restore balance and harmony to the body, mind, and spirit. Meridians are the pathways that carry vital energy or Qi throughout the body. When these pathways are blocked or disrupted, it can result in a range of physical, emotional, and mental imbalances. However, there are various techniques that can be used to address these imbalances and restore the flow of Qi through the meridians.

Acupuncture is one of the most well-known meridian techniques used to address imbalances. It involves the insertion of fine needles into specific points along the meridians to stimulate the flow of Qi. By doing so, acupuncture can help to alleviate a wide range of physical, emotional, and mental symptoms.

Another technique that can be used to address imbalances is acupressure. Acupressure is similar to acupuncture, but instead of needles, it involves applying pressure to specific points along the meridians using fingers, hands, or special devices. Acupressure can help to stimulate the flow of Qi and release any blockages or tension along the meridians.

Moxibustion is another meridian technique that can be used to address imbalances. It involves the burning of a herb called mugwort close to the skin at specific meridian points. Moxibustion can help to warm and stimulate the flow of Qi, and is often used to alleviate conditions such as colds and digestive problems.

Cupping therapy is another technique that can be used to address meridian imbalances. It involves the use of suction cups that are placed on specific meridian points to create a vacuum. The suction helps to stimulate the flow of Qi and can help to release any blockages along the meridians.

In addition to these techniques, there are also various lifestyle changes that can help to address meridian imbalances. For example, eating a healthy and balanced diet can help to support the flow of Qi and promote overall health and wellbeing. Certain foods such as ginger, garlic, and turmeric are known for their ability to promote circulation and reduce inflammation, which can help to support the flow of Qi through the meridians.

Regular exercise is also important for maintaining a healthy flow of Qi through the meridians. Exercises such as yoga, tai chi, and qigong are particularly beneficial for promoting the flow of Qi and reducing stress and tension in the body.

Meditation and mindfulness practices can also be useful for addressing meridian imbalances. These practices can help to calm the mind and reduce stress and anxiety, which can help to promote the flow of Qi through the meridians.

It's important to note that addressing meridian imbalances requires a holistic approach that takes into account the physical, emotional, and mental aspects of a person's health. By using a combination of meridian techniques and lifestyle changes, it's possible to restore balance and harmony to the body, mind, and spirit, and promote optimal health and wellbeing.

The Role of Herbs in Meridian Health

The use of herbs for medicinal purposes has been around for centuries and is deeply rooted in traditional Chinese medicine (TCM). Herbs are a natural way to support and balance the body's systems, including the meridian system. The meridian system is an essential component of TCM, which believes that energy flows through the body along these meridians. The use of herbs can help restore balance to these meridians and promote overall health and wellbeing.

The meridian system consists of twelve main meridians that are connected to specific organs in the body. Each meridian has a corresponding organ and is responsible for a specific function in the body. When the meridian system is functioning correctly, energy flows smoothly through the body, but when there is an imbalance, it can cause various physical and emotional symptoms. Herbs can be used to address these imbalances and support the meridian system.

One of the primary ways herbs are used in TCM is through herbal formulas. These formulas are a combination of various herbs that work together to address specific health concerns. Herbal formulas can be tailored to an individual's needs, and the combination of herbs is carefully selected to support the meridian system.

For example, a formula designed to support the liver meridian may include herbs such as milk thistle, dandelion root, and turmeric. These herbs help to support liver function and promote the smooth flow of energy along the liver meridian. Similarly, a formula designed to support the lung meridian may include herbs such as licorice root, ginger, and mullein. These herbs help to support lung function and promote healthy breathing.

Another way herbs can be used for meridian health is through the use of single herbs. These are individual herbs that can be used to address specific imbalances in the body. For example, ginger is known to stimulate the stomach meridian, which can help with digestive issues. Ginkgo biloba is known to support the bladder meridian and can be helpful for urinary issues.

In addition to herbal formulas and single herbs, there are also herbal teas that can be used to support the meridian system. Herbal teas are a great way to incorporate herbs into your daily routine and provide a gentle and nourishing way to support the body.

When using herbs for meridian health, it is essential to work with a qualified practitioner who can help determine the right herbs and dosages for your specific needs. Herbs can be powerful, and it is essential to use them correctly to avoid any potential side effects.

Introduction to Herbal Medicine

Herbal medicine, also known as herbalism or phytotherapy, is a traditional medicinal practice that uses plants and plant extracts to promote health and treat various illnesses. It is one of the oldest forms of medicine and has been practiced in various cultures around the world for centuries. In traditional Chinese medicine, herbs are often used to target specific meridians and support overall meridian health.

Herbs have been used for their therapeutic properties for thousands of years. Many of the most commonly used herbs in traditional medicine are derived from plants that have been found to have medicinal properties. These plants contain natural compounds that can have beneficial effects on the body. Some of the most commonly used herbs include echinacea, ginger, chamomile, and ginkgo biloba.

One of the key principles of herbal medicine is the concept of individualization. This means that treatments are tailored to each individual's unique needs and constitution. In traditional Chinese medicine, this is known as the concept of "pattern differentiation". This involves analyzing the patient's symptoms and identifying which meridians are out of balance. The appropriate herbs are then prescribed to help restore balance to the meridians and promote overall health.

There are many different ways to use herbs for meridian health. One of the most common methods is to drink herbal teas or infusions. Teas can be made using a variety of different herbs, each with their own unique benefits. For example, chamomile tea is often used to calm the mind and promote relaxation, while ginger tea can help stimulate digestion and support overall gut health.

Another way to use herbs is through topical applications. Herbal salves, ointments, and poultices can be applied directly to the skin to help treat a variety of conditions. For example, arnica is often used topically to help reduce inflammation and relieve pain.

Herbs can also be used in combination with other forms of meridian work, such as acupuncture and acupressure. In fact, many practitioners use herbal formulas in conjunction with these other modalities to help support the body's natural healing processes.

It is important to note that while herbs can be a powerful tool for supporting meridian health, they should always be used under the guidance of a trained practitioner. Herbs can interact with other medications and can cause side effects if not used properly. It is also important to ensure that any herbs used are sourced from reputable suppliers and are of high quality.

Herbs for Supporting Meridian Health

Herbs have been used for centuries to support health and wellness, and their use in traditional medicine systems continues today. In traditional Chinese medicine, herbs are often used in conjunction with acupuncture and other therapies to support meridian health. Meridians are believed to be energy pathways in the body that correspond to various organs and systems. When these pathways are blocked or out of balance, it can lead to health problems. Using herbs can be a natural and effective way to support meridian health and promote overall wellness.

One herb commonly used in traditional Chinese medicine for meridian health is ginseng. Ginseng is believed to support the lungs and spleen meridians, which are associated with immune function and digestion, respectively. Studies have also shown that ginseng may have anti-inflammatory and antioxidant properties, which can help reduce inflammation and protect against oxidative stress.

Another herb commonly used for meridian health is astragalus. Astragalus is believed to support the lung, spleen, and kidney meridians. It is often used to support the immune system and boost energy levels. Studies have shown that astragalus may also have anti-inflammatory properties, which can help reduce inflammation and support overall health.

Milk thistle is another herb commonly used in traditional medicine for meridian health. Milk thistle is believed to support the liver meridian, which is associated with detoxification and metabolism. Studies have shown that milk thistle may have hepatoprotective properties, which can help protect the liver from damage and support liver function.

Turmeric is another herb that is believed to support meridian health. Turmeric is commonly used in traditional medicine to support the spleen and stomach meridians, which are associated with digestion. Studies have shown that turmeric may have anti-inflammatory and antioxidant properties, which can help reduce inflammation and protect against oxidative stress.

In addition to these herbs, there are many other herbs that can be used to support meridian health. For example, licorice root is commonly used to support the spleen and stomach meridians, while ginger is often used to support the stomach and lung meridians. Peppermint is also believed to support the stomach meridian, and chamomile is commonly used to support the liver meridian.

When using herbs for meridian health, it is important to consult with a trained practitioner. Herbs can have side effects and interact with medications, so it is important to use them under the guidance of a knowledgeable practitioner. Additionally, herbs should be used in conjunction with other lifestyle modifications, such as diet and exercise, to support overall wellness.

The Connection Between Meridians and the Immune System

The meridian system in Traditional Chinese Medicine (TCM) is believed to play a crucial role in maintaining the body's balance and regulating the flow of energy. In TCM, it is believed that the immune system is also closely linked with the meridian system. By stimulating specific points on the meridians, the immune system can be strengthened, and the body's natural healing abilities can be enhanced.

There are 12 major meridians in TCM, and each meridian is associated with an internal organ. The immune system is closely related to the lungs, spleen, and kidneys, which are all connected to specific meridians.

The lung meridian, for example, runs from the chest down to the hand and is responsible for circulating oxygen and regulating the immune system. By stimulating specific points along the lung meridian, the immune system can be strengthened and respiratory health can be improved.

The spleen meridian runs from the big toe up the inner leg to the abdomen and is responsible for filtering blood and regulating the immune system. By stimulating specific points along the spleen meridian, the immune system can be strengthened, and the body's ability to fight off infections can be improved.

The kidney meridian runs from the foot up the inner leg to the lower abdomen and is responsible for regulating the immune system and maintaining overall health. By stimulating specific points along the kidney meridian, the immune system can be strengthened, and the body's natural healing abilities can be enhanced.

One way to stimulate these meridians and boost the immune system is through acupuncture. Acupuncture involves the insertion of thin needles into specific points along the meridians to restore the body's balance and promote healing. Acupuncture has been shown to boost the immune system by increasing the production of white blood cells and enhancing the body's natural healing abilities.

Another way to stimulate the meridians and boost the immune system is through acupressure. Acupressure involves applying pressure to specific points along the meridians using the fingers, hands, or other tools. Acupressure can help to stimulate the flow of energy along the meridians and promote the body's natural healing abilities.

In addition to acupuncture and acupressure, herbal medicine can also be used to support the immune system and stimulate the meridians. Herbs such as astragalus, echinacea, and ginseng have been used for centuries to boost the immune system and promote overall health. These herbs can be taken in supplement form or used in cooking or tea.

The Importance of a Healthy Immune System

The immune system is a complex network of cells, tissues, and organs that work together to protect the body from harmful invaders such as bacteria, viruses, and parasites. It is a vital component of overall health and wellness, as a healthy immune system can help prevent and fight off infections and diseases. Below we will explore the importance of a healthy immune system and its connection to the meridian system.

The immune system is responsible for defending the body against harmful pathogens and foreign substances that may cause harm. It is made up of various cells and tissues, including white blood cells, lymph nodes, the spleen, and bone marrow. These components work together to detect and destroy foreign invaders, while also distinguishing between harmful and harmless substances.

A healthy immune system is essential for overall health and wellbeing. It helps protect the body from infection, disease, and chronic illness. A strong immune system can also reduce the severity and duration of illnesses when they do occur.

The meridian system is a complex network of pathways that run throughout the body. It is believed to be the basis of traditional Chinese medicine and is said to be responsible for the flow of vital energy, or qi, throughout the body. The meridian system is composed of 12 major meridians, each of which corresponds to a specific organ in the body.

The meridian system and the immune system are interconnected. The meridians are thought to be responsible for the flow of energy throughout the body, including the immune system. When the flow of energy is disrupted or blocked, it can lead to imbalances in the immune system, making it more difficult for the body to fight off infections and diseases.

There are several ways to support the immune system and maintain a healthy balance in the meridian system. One of the most effective ways is through proper nutrition. Eating a balanced diet that is rich in nutrients and antioxidants can help boost the immune system and support the flow of energy throughout the body. Foods that are high in vitamin C, such as citrus fruits, berries, and leafy green vegetables, are particularly beneficial for immune health.

In addition to nutrition, exercise and stress management can also play a role in supporting immune and meridian health. Regular exercise can help improve circulation and reduce stress, which can improve the flow of energy throughout the body. Practices like yoga and meditation can also be helpful for reducing stress and promoting a healthy immune and meridian system.

There are also various natural remedies that can be used to support immune and meridian health. Herbs like echinacea, ginger, and garlic are all known for their immune-boosting properties, while essential oils like tea tree, lavender, and peppermint can be used to promote relaxation and balance in the body.

How Meridian Work Supports Immune Health

Meridian work, including acupuncture, acupressure, and other techniques, has been used for centuries to promote physical, emotional, and spiritual well-being. In recent years, research has shown that meridian work can also have a positive impact on the immune system. The immune system is responsible for defending the body against infections, diseases, and other harmful agents. When the immune system is weakened or compromised, the body becomes more susceptible to illnesses and diseases. Below we will explore the connection between meridian work and immune health, and how meridian work can support the immune system.

The immune system is a complex network of cells, tissues, and organs that work together to protect the body against harmful pathogens, such as bacteria, viruses, and fungi. The immune system also plays a key role in preventing the growth and spread of cancer cells. When the immune system is functioning properly, it can recognize and destroy harmful pathogens before they can cause harm to the body. However, when the immune system is weakened or compromised, it may not be able to effectively fight off these harmful agents, which can lead to infections and illnesses.

Meridian work can help support the immune system in several ways. One way is by improving circulation. The meridians are channels of energy that run throughout the body. When these meridians become blocked or stagnant, it can disrupt the flow of energy and lead to imbalances in the body. By stimulating the meridians through acupuncture, acupressure, or other techniques, it can help improve circulation and restore balance to the body. This improved circulation can help deliver nutrients and oxygen to the cells and tissues of the body, which can support the immune system.

Another way that meridian work can support the immune system is by reducing stress. Stress can have a negative impact on the immune system by suppressing its function. When the body is under stress, it produces cortisol, a hormone that can weaken the immune system. By reducing stress through meridian work, it can help improve the function of the immune system. Acupuncture, in particular, has been shown to reduce stress levels by stimulating the release of endorphins, which are the body's natural painkillers and mood elevators.

Meridian work can also help stimulate the production of white blood cells, which are the body's primary defense against infections and diseases. White blood cells are produced in the bone marrow and circulate throughout the body, seeking out and destroying harmful pathogens. Studies have shown that acupuncture and acupressure can help increase the production of white blood cells, which can help strengthen the immune system.

Certain acupuncture points are also believed to have a direct impact on the immune system. For example, the point known as "Zusanli" or ST36, which is located on the stomach meridian, has been shown to stimulate the production of T-cells, which are a type of white blood cell that play a key role in the immune response. Another point, known as "Guanyuan" or CV4, which is located on the conception vessel meridian, has been shown to stimulate the production of antibodies, which are proteins that help fight off infections and diseases.

In addition to meridian work, there are several lifestyle factors that can help support the immune system. These include getting enough sleep, exercising regularly, eating a healthy diet, managing stress, and avoiding smoking and excessive alcohol consumption. By incorporating these lifestyle factors into your daily routine, along with meridian work, you can help support your immune system and reduce your risk of infections and illnesses.

Meridian Health and Sleep

Meridians are a key component of traditional Chinese medicine (TCM) and are believed to be the pathways through which life energy, or Qi, flows through the body. There are 12 major meridians, each associated with a specific organ or system in the body. The health of these meridians is crucial for the optimal functioning of the body, including proper sleep.

Sleep is an essential aspect of human health, and a lack of quality sleep can lead to a range of physical and mental health issues. Studies have shown that the meridian system plays a significant role in regulating sleep patterns and improving sleep quality.

According to TCM, each meridian is associated with a specific time of day when its energy is at its peak. For example, the Liver meridian is most active between 1-3 am, while the Lung meridian is most active between 3-5 am. By stimulating the appropriate meridians during their peak times, it is believed that one can improve their sleep quality.

One way to stimulate the meridians is through acupuncture. Acupuncture involves the insertion of fine needles into specific points along the meridians to balance the flow of Qi. Research has shown that acupuncture can improve sleep quality and duration by regulating the production of neurotransmitters such as melatonin and serotonin, which are involved in regulating sleep patterns.

In addition to acupuncture, there are other meridian-based practices that can improve sleep. For example, acupressure involves applying pressure to specific meridian points with the fingers or massage tools to stimulate the flow of Qi. This can be done at any time of day or night, making it a convenient option for those looking to improve their sleep.

Another meridian-based practice that can improve sleep is Qigong. Qigong involves slow, gentle movements and breathing exercises designed to balance the flow of Qi in the body. Research has shown that regular Qigong practice can improve sleep quality and duration.

In addition to these practices, there are also lifestyle factors that can affect meridian health and, consequently, sleep quality. For example, stress can lead to meridian imbalances, which can disrupt sleep patterns. Engaging in stress-reducing activities such as meditation, yoga, or mindfulness practices can help to balance the meridians and improve sleep quality.

Diet is also important for meridian health and sleep. In TCM, each organ system is associated with a specific flavor, and consuming foods with those flavors is believed to nourish the corresponding meridian. For example, the Liver meridian is associated with the sour flavor, while the Heart meridian is associated with the bitter flavor. Consuming foods with these flavors can help to balance the corresponding meridians and improve sleep quality.

The Importance of Quality Sleep

Sleep is a vital aspect of our daily lives, as it is the time when our bodies and minds rest and recover from the day's activities. However, many people struggle with getting enough quality sleep, which can have negative effects on their overall health and well-being. Below we will explore the importance of quality sleep in relation to the twelve major meridians.

The meridians are channels that run throughout the body, according to traditional Chinese medicine (TCM). They are believed to be pathways for the flow of vital energy, known as qi, which nourishes and sustains all the body's systems. Each meridian is associated with a specific organ system and is believed to affect various aspects of our physical and emotional health.

One of the meridians that is particularly important for sleep is the heart meridian. The heart is responsible for regulating the body's circadian rhythms, which control our sleep-wake cycles. When the heart meridian is imbalanced, it can lead to insomnia, restless sleep, and other sleep disturbances.

The liver meridian is also important for sleep, as it is responsible for detoxifying the body and regulating the flow of energy throughout the body. An imbalance in the liver meridian can cause irritability, anxiety, and difficulty falling asleep.

The lung meridian is another meridian that plays a role in sleep, as it is responsible for regulating the breath and promoting relaxation. An imbalance in the lung meridian can lead to shallow breathing, which can disrupt sleep and cause fatigue.

The kidney meridian is also important for sleep, as it is responsible for regulating the body's water balance and promoting relaxation. An imbalance in the kidney meridian can lead to insomnia, night sweats, and other sleep disturbances.

In addition to the specific meridians that affect sleep, TCM also recognizes the importance of overall balance and harmony in the body. When the body's energy is balanced and flowing smoothly, it is easier to achieve quality sleep and maintain good health.

There are several techniques that can be used to support meridian health and promote quality sleep. Acupuncture is one such technique, which involves the insertion of fine needles into specific points on the body to stimulate the flow of energy and promote relaxation. Acupuncture can be particularly effective for addressing imbalances in the heart, liver, lung, and kidney meridians.

Moxibustion is another technique that can be used to support meridian health and promote quality sleep. Moxibustion involves the burning of dried mugwort on specific acupuncture points to stimulate the flow of energy and promote relaxation. Moxibustion can be particularly effective for addressing imbalances in the kidney and liver meridians.

Cupping is also a technique that can be used to support meridian health and promote quality sleep. Cupping involves the placement of glass or plastic cups on specific points on the body to create a suction effect that stimulates the flow of energy and promotes relaxation. Cupping can be particularly effective for addressing imbalances in the lung and heart meridians.

In addition to these techniques, there are also lifestyle changes that can be made to support meridian health and promote quality sleep. Eating a balanced diet that includes foods that support the meridians, such as leafy greens for the liver meridian and warm, nourishing foods for the kidney meridian, can be helpful. Regular exercise, stress management techniques, and a consistent sleep schedule can also support meridian health and promote quality sleep.

How Meridian Work Can Improve Sleep

Sleep is an essential aspect of our lives, and lack of it can negatively impact our overall health and wellbeing. While there are many different factors that can affect our sleep, meridian work is one approach that can help improve sleep quality and duration. Below we will explore the connection between meridian work and sleep, and how meridian work can improve sleep.

What are Meridians?

Meridians are channels or pathways that run throughout our bodies, connecting our internal organs and tissues. According to traditional Chinese medicine, the flow of energy or life force, known as Qi (pronounced "chee"), travels through these meridians. The Qi flow can become blocked or unbalanced, leading to a variety of physical, emotional, and mental health issues.

The Twelve Major Meridians

There are twelve major meridians in the body, each associated with a specific internal organ or organ system. These meridians include the lung meridian, large intestine meridian, stomach meridian, spleen meridian, heart meridian, small intestine meridian, bladder meridian, kidney meridian, pericardium meridian, triple warmer meridian, gallbladder meridian, and liver meridian.

How Meridian Work Can Improve Sleep

Meridian work involves techniques that stimulate the flow of Qi through the meridians, promoting balance and improving overall health. Here are some ways that meridian work can help improve sleep:

Reducing Stress and Anxiety

Stress and anxiety can interfere with sleep, making it difficult to fall asleep or stay asleep. By stimulating the meridians associated with relaxation, such as the heart, pericardium, and liver meridians, meridian work can help reduce stress and anxiety levels, promoting a more peaceful and restful sleep.

Balancing Energy

Meridian work aims to balance the flow of Qi through the meridians, promoting overall health and wellbeing. When the Qi flow is unbalanced, it can lead to physical, emotional, and mental health issues, including sleep disturbances. By addressing the underlying imbalances in the meridians, meridian work can help improve sleep quality and duration.

Regulating the Circadian Rhythm

The circadian rhythm is our internal biological clock that regulates our sleep-wake cycle. Disruptions to the circadian rhythm, such as jet lag or shift work, can negatively impact our sleep. Meridian work can help regulate the circadian rhythm by stimulating the meridians associated with sleep, such as the heart, pericardium, and kidney meridians.

Addressing Underlying Health Issues

Chronic health issues can interfere with sleep, making it difficult to get the rest we need. Meridian work can address underlying health issues by stimulating the meridians associated with specific organs or organ systems. For example, stimulating the lung meridian can help alleviate respiratory issues that may be interfering with sleep.

Promoting Relaxation and Calm

Meridian work techniques such as acupressure, acupuncture, and qigong involve gentle pressure, needles, or movements that promote relaxation and calm. By stimulating the meridians associated with relaxation, such as the heart and pericardium meridians, meridian work can help promote a sense of calm and relaxation that can lead to a more restful sleep.

Meridian Health and Aging

Meridians are channels or pathways that run through the body, carrying the flow of qi (pronounced chee), the vital energy that sustains life. There are twelve major meridians that are linked to specific organs and functions within the body. These meridians are responsible for maintaining the balance of energy in the body and any blockages or imbalances in them can lead to a range of physical and emotional health problems. As we age, our meridians can become blocked or weakened, affecting our overall health and wellbeing. Below we will explore the importance of maintaining healthy meridians as we age and how meridian work can support healthy aging.

As we age, the flow of qi in our meridians can become disrupted, leading to blockages and imbalances that can manifest as a variety of physical and emotional symptoms. These may include fatigue, pain, stiffness, insomnia, depression, and anxiety. Additionally, as we age, our organs can become less efficient, which can further affect the flow of qi through our meridians.

One of the key ways to maintain healthy meridians as we age is through regular meridian work, which can include acupuncture, acupressure, massage, and other meridian-based therapies. These therapies aim to restore the flow of qi through the meridians, removing any blockages and imbalances and promoting overall health and wellbeing.

Acupuncture, for example, involves the insertion of thin needles into specific points on the meridians, which helps to stimulate the flow of qi and promote healing. Acupressure, on the other hand, involves the application of pressure to these same points, either with the hands or with specialized tools, to achieve similar effects. Massage, which can include both meridian massage and more general forms of massage, can also help to promote the flow of qi and improve overall health and wellbeing.

In addition to these therapies, there are also a number of other ways to support healthy meridians as we age. These may include practicing yoga, tai chi, or other forms of exercise that focus on breath and movement, as well as eating a healthy, balanced diet that includes a variety of nutrient-rich foods.

Certain herbs and supplements can also be beneficial for maintaining healthy meridians as we age. For example, ginseng, which has been used in traditional Chinese medicine for thousands of years, is believed to promote overall health and wellbeing, as well as improve cognitive function, immune function, and cardiovascular health. Other herbs, such as ginger, turmeric, and green tea, have also been shown to have anti-inflammatory and antioxidant effects, which can help to support healthy aging.

It is important to note that while meridian work and other therapies can be beneficial for promoting healthy aging, they should not be used in place of other medical treatments. If you are experiencing any health concerns, it is important to consult with a healthcare professional before beginning any new therapies or treatments.

The Aging Process and Its Effects on Meridians

The aging process is a natural part of life that affects all living organisms. As we age, our bodies undergo a series of changes that can have significant effects on our overall health and wellbeing. One area where these changes can have a particularly pronounced impact is the meridian system.

The meridian system is a network of pathways that connect various parts of the body and facilitate the flow of vital energy, or Qi. These pathways are believed to correspond to specific organs and body systems, and imbalances in the meridian system can lead to a range of physical and emotional symptoms.

As we age, our meridian system may become less efficient at regulating the flow of Qi. This can be due to a variety of factors, including changes in hormone levels, decreased physical activity, and exposure to environmental toxins. Over time, these imbalances can lead to a range of health problems, including chronic pain, fatigue, and weakened immune function.

One common age-related meridian imbalance is a deficiency in the kidney meridian. The kidney meridian is associated with the body's vital energy reserves, and as we age, these reserves may become depleted. This can lead to symptoms such as lower back pain, fatigue, and a weakened immune system.

Another common meridian imbalance associated with aging is a deficiency in the spleen meridian. The spleen meridian is responsible for regulating digestion and nutrient absorption, and as we age, it may become less efficient at these functions. This can lead to symptoms such as bloating, gas, and poor appetite.

Despite these challenges, there are many ways to support meridian health as we age. One important step is to maintain a healthy lifestyle, including a balanced diet, regular exercise, and stress-reducing activities such as meditation or yoga.

In addition, targeted meridian work can be an effective way to address specific imbalances and support overall health and wellbeing. This may involve techniques such as acupressure, acupuncture, or herbal remedies.

Acupressure is a form of meridian work that involves applying pressure to specific points along the meridian pathways. This can help to stimulate the flow of Qi, relieve tension and pain, and promote overall balance and wellbeing. Acupuncture, which involves the insertion of fine needles into specific meridian points, is another effective technique for supporting meridian health.

Herbal remedies can also be effective for addressing specific meridian imbalances. For example, ginseng is a popular herb used to support kidney meridian health, while ginger can help to support the spleen meridian. Other herbs, such as turmeric, chamomile, and ashwagandha, may also have beneficial effects on the meridian system.

In addition to these targeted interventions, it's also important to prioritize rest and relaxation as we age. Getting enough sleep, taking breaks when needed, and engaging in activities that bring joy and fulfillment can all help to support meridian health and overall wellbeing.

How to Support Meridian Health as We Age

As we age, our bodies undergo various changes, including changes to our meridian system. The meridians are a network of energy pathways that run through our bodies, and when they are functioning optimally, we experience good health and well-being. However, as we age, these pathways can become blocked or imbalanced, leading to a range of physical and emotional issues. Below we will explore how to support meridian health as we age.

One of the most important things we can do to support our meridian health as we age is to stay active. Regular exercise is crucial for keeping our meridian pathways open and flowing freely. Even gentle exercises like tai chi or yoga can be incredibly beneficial for promoting meridian health. These practices help to improve circulation, stimulate the flow of qi (life force energy), and promote relaxation, all of which can help to support the proper functioning of our meridians.

Another important factor in maintaining meridian health as we age is proper nutrition. Our bodies require a balance of nutrients to function properly, and this is especially true for the meridian system. Eating a diet rich in whole, nutrient-dense foods can help to support the health of our meridians. This includes foods like fruits, vegetables, whole grains, lean proteins, and healthy fats. Additionally, there are certain foods that are specifically beneficial for supporting meridian health, such as ginger, garlic, turmeric, and green tea.

Along with exercise and nutrition, it is also important to practice stress management techniques to support meridian health as we age. Stress can have a significant impact on our meridian system, leading to blockages and imbalances. Practices like meditation, deep breathing, and mindfulness can help to reduce stress and promote relaxation, which can in turn support the proper functioning of our meridians.

Another way to support meridian health as we age is through regular meridian massage or acupuncture treatments. These practices involve stimulating specific points along the meridian pathways, which can help to clear blockages and promote the free flow of qi. Regular treatments can be incredibly beneficial for maintaining meridian health and preventing imbalances from developing.

Finally, it is important to stay connected with our bodies and to pay attention to any signs of imbalances or blockages in our meridian system. This includes being aware of physical symptoms like pain, stiffness, or numbness, as well as emotional symptoms like anxiety, depression, or irritability. By being aware of these signs, we can take proactive steps to address any imbalances before they become more serious.

The Role of Meridians in Pain Management

Meridians are an essential part of Traditional Chinese Medicine (TCM), which is based on the idea that the human body has a network of channels or pathways called meridians. Meridians are thought to carry energy or qi (pronounced "chee") throughout the body, and any blockages or imbalances in the meridian system can cause pain, illness, and disease. The concept of meridians is used in various healing modalities, including acupuncture, acupressure, cupping, and moxibustion, and plays a crucial role in pain management.

Pain is a common problem that affects millions of people worldwide. It can be caused by many factors, including injury, illness, or chronic conditions such as arthritis. Pain can be acute or chronic, and it can affect people physically, emotionally, and mentally. Many people turn to pain medications to manage their pain, but these drugs can have harmful side effects and may not be effective in treating all types of pain. Meridian-based therapies offer a natural and holistic approach to pain management that can be both safe and effective.

The meridian system is thought to be a complex network of channels that carry energy throughout the body. According to TCM theory, when there is an imbalance in the flow of energy in the meridians, pain and illness can occur. The meridian system is thought to be connected to the body's internal organs, and each meridian is associated with a particular organ system. For example, the liver meridian is thought to be associated with the liver and gallbladder, and the heart meridian with the heart and circulatory system.

One of the most well-known meridian-based therapies for pain management is acupuncture. Acupuncture is an ancient Chinese healing modality that involves the insertion of thin needles into specific points along the meridians to stimulate the flow of energy and restore balance. Acupuncture has been used for centuries to treat a wide range of conditions, including pain, and is becoming increasingly popular in Western countries.

Another meridian-based therapy that can help with pain management is acupressure. Acupressure is similar to acupuncture but involves the application of pressure to specific points on the meridians using the hands, fingers, or other objects. Acupressure can be used to relieve pain, reduce stress and tension, and promote relaxation.

Cupping therapy is another meridian-based therapy that can be effective for pain management. Cupping involves the use of special cups that are placed on the skin to create a suction effect. The cups are typically left in place for several minutes and can help to increase blood flow, reduce inflammation, and relieve pain.

Moxibustion is another meridian-based therapy that can be used for pain management. Moxibustion involves the burning of dried mugwort leaves over specific points along the meridians to stimulate the flow of energy and promote healing. Moxibustion can be used to relieve pain, reduce inflammation, and promote overall health and well-being.

In addition to these meridian-based therapies, lifestyle changes can also help to support meridian health and manage pain. Exercise, for example, can help to improve circulation, reduce inflammation, and promote overall health and well-being. Yoga and tai chi, in particular, can be beneficial for people with chronic pain as they help to promote relaxation, reduce stress, and improve flexibility.

Diet can also play a role in meridian health and pain management. According to TCM theory, certain foods can help to support the meridian system and promote overall health and well-being. Foods that are thought to be beneficial for the meridians include ginger, turmeric, garlic, and onions.

Understanding Chronic Pain

Chronic pain is a complex and often debilitating condition that affects millions of people around the world. It can result from a wide range of conditions, including injuries, illnesses, and chronic diseases. While acute pain is a normal response to injury or tissue damage, chronic pain is a persistent, ongoing pain that can last for months or even years. Chronic pain can have a significant impact on a person's quality of life, affecting their ability to work, participate in activities they enjoy, and even perform daily tasks.

The causes of chronic pain are varied and can include structural issues, such as a herniated disc, nerve damage, or arthritis. In some cases, chronic pain can also result from psychological factors, such as depression, anxiety, or stress. While there are many treatment options available for chronic pain, including medications, physical therapy, and surgery, many people are turning to alternative therapies, such as acupuncture, massage, and meridian work, to manage their pain.

Meridian work is a form of traditional Chinese medicine that involves manipulating the body's energy pathways, or meridians, to restore balance and promote healing. The meridians are believed to be channels that carry energy, or qi, throughout the body. When the meridians become blocked or imbalanced, it can lead to a wide range of physical and emotional symptoms, including pain.

There are 12 major meridians in the body, each associated with specific organs and functions. These meridians are named after the organs they are associated with, such as the liver meridian, kidney meridian, and lung meridian. Each meridian has a different pathway through the body and is connected to specific acupuncture points.

When a person experiences chronic pain, it is often an indication that there is an imbalance or blockage in one or more of the meridians. By working to restore balance and unblock these pathways, meridian work can help to reduce pain and improve overall health and well-being.

One of the primary ways that meridian work can help to manage chronic pain is by promoting the body's natural healing processes. By stimulating specific acupuncture points along the affected meridians, meridian work can help to increase blood flow, reduce inflammation, and release endorphins, the body's natural painkillers.

In addition to promoting healing, meridian work can also help to address the underlying emotional and psychological factors that often accompany chronic pain. According to traditional Chinese medicine, emotional imbalances, such as stress, anxiety, and depression, can lead to blockages in the meridians and contribute to chronic pain. By addressing these emotional factors, meridian work can help to reduce pain and improve overall well-being.

There are many different types of meridian work that can be used to manage chronic pain, including acupuncture, acupressure, and meridian massage. Each of these techniques works by stimulating specific acupuncture points along the meridians, either through the use of needles, pressure, or massage.

Acupuncture involves inserting thin needles into the skin at specific points along the meridians. This can help to stimulate the flow of energy and promote healing. Acupressure, on the other hand, involves applying pressure to specific acupuncture points using the fingers, hands, or special tools. This can help to release tension and improve blood flow, reducing pain and promoting healing.

Meridian massage is another popular form of meridian work that can be used to manage chronic pain. This technique involves massaging the body along the meridians, using a combination of pressure and stretching to release tension and promote healing.

How Meridian Work Can Help Manage Pain

Meridian work, also known as meridian therapy or energy medicine, is a form of alternative therapy that aims to balance the body's energy flow through the stimulation of specific points along the meridians, or energy channels, in the body. This type of therapy has been used for thousands of years in traditional Chinese medicine and has recently gained popularity as a complementary approach to pain management.

Pain is a common symptom experienced by people of all ages and can be caused by a variety of factors, including injury, inflammation, or chronic conditions such as arthritis or fibromyalgia. Chronic pain, which is defined as pain lasting for more than 3 months, can have a significant impact on an individual's physical, emotional, and social well-being. Conventional treatments for pain management include medications, physical therapy, and surgery. However, these treatments may not always be effective or may come with unwanted side effects.

Meridian work offers a non-invasive, drug-free approach to pain management. According to traditional Chinese medicine, pain is caused by an imbalance in the body's energy flow. By stimulating the appropriate points along the meridians, meridian work can help restore balance and alleviate pain.

There are twelve major meridians in the body, each associated with a specific organ system. These meridians run through the body in a continuous circuit, connecting different areas and systems. Each meridian has specific points that can be stimulated to help balance energy flow and alleviate pain.

Acupressure and acupuncture are two common techniques used in meridian work. Acupressure involves applying pressure to specific points along the meridians using fingers, palms, or elbows. Acupuncture involves the insertion of thin needles into the skin at specific points along the meridians. Both techniques aim to stimulate the body's natural healing response and promote balance in energy flow.

Research has shown that meridian work may be effective in managing various types of pain, including low back pain, neck pain, and osteoarthritis. In a systematic review of randomized controlled trials, researchers found that acupuncture was more effective than no treatment or sham acupuncture for chronic pain. Another study found that acupressure was effective in reducing pain and improving sleep in patients with chronic low back pain.

In addition to acupressure and acupuncture, there are other meridian-based techniques that may help manage pain. These include qigong, tai chi, and meridian massage. Qigong and tai chi are gentle exercises that involve movements, breathing techniques, and meditation. These exercises aim to promote balance in energy flow and improve overall well-being. Meridian massage involves the application of pressure to specific points along the meridians using massage techniques. This type of massage aims to release tension and promote relaxation.

In addition to its potential benefits in pain management, meridian work may also have other health benefits. Studies have shown that acupuncture and acupressure may help reduce anxiety, depression, and stress. Qigong and tai chi have been shown to improve balance, flexibility, and overall physical function in older adults.

Integrating Meridian Work into Daily Life

Meridian work is a holistic approach to health that has been used for centuries in traditional Chinese medicine. It involves working with the body's energy pathways, or meridians, to promote balance and vitality. While meridian work may have been viewed as esoteric or unfamiliar to many in the West, it is gaining popularity as people seek natural and effective ways to support their health and well-being. One of the most significant benefits of meridian work is that it can be easily integrated into daily life, allowing individuals to practice self-care and cultivate greater mind-body awareness.

To understand how meridian work can be integrated into daily life, it is essential to first understand the basics of meridian theory. In traditional Chinese medicine, the body is believed to be composed of a system of energy channels or meridians through which life force or "qi" flows. Each meridian is associated with a specific organ system and corresponds to a different aspect of physical, emotional, and spiritual health. According to traditional Chinese medicine, when the flow of qi is disrupted or blocked, it can lead to physical or emotional imbalances, illness, or pain.

One way to support meridian health is through acupuncture, a practice that involves inserting fine needles into specific points along the meridians to stimulate the flow of qi. However, there are other ways to work with the meridians that do not require needles or the assistance of a practitioner. These include techniques such as acupressure, meridian tapping, and qigong.

Acupressure involves using gentle pressure with the fingers or hands to stimulate specific points along the meridians. By applying pressure to these points, known as acupoints, one can help release blockages and promote the flow of qi. This technique can be easily integrated into daily life by simply using your fingers to apply pressure to acupoints throughout the day. For example, if you are experiencing stress or tension, you could apply pressure to the "third eye" acupoint located between the eyebrows to help calm the mind and promote relaxation.

Meridian tapping, also known as Emotional Freedom Technique (EFT), is another method of working with the meridians that can be done easily and quickly at any time. It involves tapping specific acupoints while focusing on a particular issue or emotion. By tapping on these points while acknowledging and accepting the issue or emotion, individuals can release negative energy and promote a more positive mindset. For example, if you are feeling anxious or overwhelmed, you could tap on the "karate chop" point on the side of the hand while repeating a calming affirmation such as "I am calm and peaceful."

Qigong, an ancient practice that combines movement, breathwork, and visualization, is another way to support meridian health. Qigong exercises are designed to help cultivate and balance the flow of qi in the body, promoting physical, emotional, and spiritual well-being. Practicing qigong regularly can help individuals become more in tune with their bodies, promoting greater awareness and mindfulness throughout the day.

In addition to these specific techniques, there are many other ways to support meridian health in daily life. These include:

Eating a balanced diet that supports the specific organ systems associated with each meridian. For example, consuming foods that support the digestive system can help promote the health of the stomach and spleen meridians.

Practicing good sleep hygiene to promote rest and rejuvenation of the body's energy systems.

Engaging in regular exercise or movement that promotes the flow of qi, such as yoga or tai chi.

Spending time in nature to help ground and balance the body's energy systems.

Tips for Incorporating Meridian Practices

Meridian practices, such as acupuncture, acupressure, and qigong, have been used for centuries to promote physical, emotional, and spiritual health. These practices work by stimulating specific points along the body's meridian pathways, which are believed to be channels of energy flow. While these practices can be beneficial on their own, incorporating them into your daily routine can further enhance their benefits. Here are some tips for incorporating meridian practices into your daily life:

Start with simple practices: If you are new to meridian practices, start with simple exercises that can be easily integrated into your daily routine. For example, you can practice deep breathing, stretching, or gentle movements such as qigong or tai chi.

Incorporate meridian points into your daily routine: You can stimulate meridian points throughout the day by pressing on specific points on your hands, feet, and ears. For example, pressing on the point between your thumb and index finger can help relieve headaches and stimulate digestion.

Practice mindfulness: Mindfulness meditation can help you tune into your body and become more aware of your meridian pathways. You can practice mindfulness by focusing on your breath, paying attention to sensations in your body, and observing your thoughts without judgment.

Use essential oils: Essential oils can be used to enhance the benefits of meridian practices. For example, peppermint oil can help stimulate the digestive system, while lavender oil can help promote relaxation and sleep.

Seek professional guidance: If you are interested in incorporating meridian practices into your daily routine, consider seeking guidance from a trained professional. A licensed acupuncturist or qigong instructor can help you develop a personalized practice that is tailored to your specific needs.

Practice consistently: Like any other form of self-care, meridian practices require consistency to be effective. Set aside time each day to practice, even if it is only for a few minutes.

Listen to your body: As you begin to incorporate meridian practices into your daily routine, pay attention to how your body responds. If a certain practice feels uncomfortable or does not resonate with you, listen to your body and adjust your practice accordingly.

Incorporating meridian practices into your daily routine can help promote physical, emotional, and spiritual health. By starting with simple practices, incorporating meridian points throughout your day, practicing mindfulness, using essential oils, seeking professional guidance, practicing consistently, and listening to your body, you can enhance the benefits of these ancient practices and live a more balanced and fulfilling life.

Creating a Personalized Meridian Routine

The meridian system in Traditional Chinese Medicine (TCM) is a complex network of energy channels that run throughout the body, connecting various organs and tissues. It is believed that the smooth flow of energy or qi through these meridians is essential for maintaining physical and emotional health. A meridian routine is a set of practices that aim to balance and harmonize the flow of qi in the body. Below we will explore the benefits of a personalized meridian routine and how to create one for yourself.

Benefits of a Personalized Meridian Routine

A personalized meridian routine can offer numerous benefits for your physical and emotional well-being. Here are some of the key benefits of incorporating meridian practices into your daily routine:

Improved energy flow: A personalized meridian routine can help improve the flow of qi in your body. When energy is flowing smoothly through the meridians, you may experience greater physical vitality and mental clarity.

Reduced stress and anxiety: Certain meridian practices, such as acupressure or meditation, can help reduce stress and anxiety. This can be particularly beneficial for those who experience chronic stress or anxiety.

Better sleep: Many meridian practices, including acupuncture, acupressure, and certain meditations, can help improve sleep quality. This is especially important for those who struggle with sleep disorders or insomnia.

Reduced pain and inflammation: Certain meridian practices, such as acupuncture and acupressure, have been shown to help reduce pain and inflammation. This can be particularly beneficial for those who suffer from chronic pain conditions.

Creating a Personalized Meridian Routine

Creating a personalized meridian routine involves a combination of self-exploration and experimentation. Here are some tips for creating a routine that works for you:

Set an intention: Before you begin, it can be helpful to set an intention for your meridian routine. What do you hope to achieve? What are your goals? This can help you stay motivated and focused as you explore different practices.

Start small: If you are new to meridian practices, it's important to start small and gradually build up. You don't need to do everything at once. Start with one or two practices and gradually add more as you feel comfortable.

Experiment with different practices: There are many different meridian practices to choose from, including acupuncture, acupressure, meridian stretches, and meditation. Experiment with different practices and find the ones that resonate with you.

Create a schedule: Once you have identified the practices that work for you, create a schedule that you can stick to. This might involve practicing certain techniques at the same time each day or setting aside specific times during the week for longer practices.

Be patient: It can take time to see the benefits of a meridian routine. Be patient and stick with it. Over time, you may notice improvements in your physical and emotional well-being.

The Future of Meridian Research

The meridian system has been a fundamental concept in traditional Chinese medicine (TCM) for thousands of years. It refers to the network of energy pathways that circulate throughout the body, connecting organs and other body parts. The meridians are believed to be responsible for the flow of vital energy or Qi, which is essential for overall health and well-being. In recent years, the meridian system has gained interest in the Western world, leading to increased research and exploration. Below we will discuss the current and future state of meridian research.

To date, much of the research on the meridian system has been conducted in the context of TCM. While this research has provided valuable insights into the meridian system and its potential health benefits, it has been criticized for a lack of scientific rigor and standardization. This has limited its applicability to the broader medical community and has been a major barrier to further exploration.

However, recent developments in technology and scientific methodology have opened up new avenues for meridian research. For example, advanced imaging techniques such as magnetic resonance imaging (MRI) and positron emission tomography (PET) can now be used to visualize and map the meridian system in detail. This has led to a better understanding of the meridian pathways and their relationship to various organs and body functions.

Furthermore, recent studies have explored the physiological mechanisms underlying the meridian system. For example, researchers have investigated the role of the nervous system in the transmission of energy along the meridians. They have also explored the connection between the meridians and the body's fascial network, which is a complex web of connective tissue that surrounds and supports muscles, bones, and organs.

Another area of research that shows promise is the use of meridian-based therapies for various health conditions. For example, acupuncture, which is based on the principles of the meridian system, has been shown to be effective for the treatment of chronic pain, headaches, and other conditions. Other meridian-based therapies, such as acupressure, reflexology, and meridian massage, have also been explored for their potential health benefits.

Despite these advances, much more research is needed to fully understand the meridian system and its potential health benefits. In particular, there is a need for more standardized and rigorous research methods to ensure that the findings are reproducible and can be translated into clinical practice.

In the future, it is likely that meridian research will continue to focus on the physiological mechanisms underlying the meridian system, as well as the potential health benefits of meridian-based therapies. This will require collaboration between researchers in different fields, including traditional medicine, neuroscience, and engineering.

It is also possible that new technologies and techniques will be developed to further explore the meridian system. For example, researchers may develop non-invasive techniques for stimulating the meridians or tracking the flow of energy along the pathways.

Another area of future research is the relationship between the meridian system and other aspects of health and wellness, such as nutrition, exercise, and mental health. Researchers may explore how these factors impact the meridian system and how meridian-based therapies can be integrated into a broader approach to health and wellness.

Current Research and Findings

The meridian system, a network of energy pathways in the body, has been the focus of research for centuries. Ancient Chinese medicine first documented the meridian system, and it has since been studied by scientists and researchers around the world. In recent years, there has been an increase in research on the meridian system, leading to exciting new findings and possibilities for the future.

One of the primary areas of research on the meridian system has been in acupuncture, a traditional Chinese medicine practice that involves inserting needles into specific points along the meridians to stimulate healing. Studies have shown that acupuncture can be effective in treating a variety of conditions, including chronic pain, nausea, and depression. Researchers have also found that acupuncture can stimulate the release of endorphins, the body's natural painkillers, and can improve blood flow to affected areas.

In addition to acupuncture, there has been growing interest in other forms of meridian therapy, such as acupressure and meridian massage. These practices involve applying pressure or massage to specific meridian points, and research has shown that they can be effective in reducing pain, promoting relaxation, and improving overall health.

Another area of research on the meridian system has been in the use of meridian imaging techniques, such as infrared thermography and electrodermal screening, to assess meridian function and diagnose health conditions. These techniques involve measuring changes in skin temperature or electrical conductivity at specific meridian points, and have shown promise in detecting imbalances or blockages in the meridian system.

Research has also explored the relationship between the meridian system and other aspects of health, such as the immune system, digestive system, and nervous system. Studies have shown that meridian therapy can stimulate the immune system, promote healthy digestion, and reduce stress and anxiety.

One particularly exciting area of research on the meridian system has been in the use of bioelectromagnetic therapy, which involves applying low-level electromagnetic fields to the body to stimulate healing. Research has shown that electromagnetic fields can affect the flow of energy along the meridians, and may have a beneficial effect on a variety of health conditions, including pain, inflammation, and neurological disorders.

While there have been many promising findings in meridian research, there is still much to be learned about the meridian system and its role in health and disease. As researchers continue to explore this complex system, it is likely that new discoveries will emerge, leading to new and more effective approaches to health and wellness.

The Potential for Future Developments in Meridian Health

Meridian health is a crucial aspect of overall health and wellbeing. Meridians, also known as energy channels, play a significant role in Traditional Chinese Medicine (TCM) and acupuncture. In TCM, meridians are believed to be channels through which energy, or Qi, flows throughout the body. When these channels are blocked or imbalanced, it can lead to a variety of physical and emotional health issues. However, through meridian work, such as acupuncture, acupressure, and meridian massage, these imbalances can be addressed and optimal health can be achieved.

While meridian work has been around for thousands of years, current research is shedding new light on its potential benefits and future developments. Recent studies have shown that meridian work can have a positive impact on a variety of health conditions, including chronic pain, anxiety, and insomnia. In addition, advancements in technology and research techniques are allowing for a more detailed understanding of the meridian system and how it interacts with other systems in the body.

One area of potential future development is the use of meridian work in conjunction with Western medicine. While TCM and Western medicine have traditionally been viewed as separate practices, there is increasing interest in combining the two to create a more holistic approach to healthcare. For example, some studies have shown that acupuncture can be an effective treatment for chronic pain, and it may be used in conjunction with other Western treatments to provide patients with a comprehensive approach to pain management.

In addition, advancements in technology are allowing for a better understanding of the meridian system and how it relates to other systems in the body. For example, researchers are exploring the relationship between meridians and the nervous system. One study found that acupuncture can activate the brain's reward system, which may explain its ability to reduce pain and improve mood. Other studies are investigating the relationship between meridians and the lymphatic system, which plays a crucial role in immune function.

Another area of potential future development is the use of meridian work for preventative care. While meridian work is often used to address existing health issues, it may also be useful for maintaining optimal health and preventing future health problems. For example, regular acupuncture treatments may help to balance the body's energy flow and reduce the risk of imbalances that can lead to health issues. Similarly, meridian massage can be used as a preventative measure to maintain optimal energy flow and promote overall health and wellbeing.

The Importance of Meridian Health

The human body is an intricate system of interconnecting parts, each responsible for a specific function. One of the most vital systems is the meridian system, which is responsible for the flow of energy throughout the body. Meridians are pathways that carry life force energy or "qi" throughout the body. These meridians are connected to various organs and functions in the body, and when they become blocked or imbalanced, it can lead to physical and emotional discomfort. Therefore, it is crucial to maintain the health of these meridians to promote overall well-being.

The meridian system is composed of 12 main meridians, each associated with specific organs and functions. These meridians run vertically through the body and are mirrored on each side of the body. When these meridians are functioning correctly, they allow for the smooth flow of qi throughout the body, resulting in optimal health. However, when these meridians become blocked or imbalanced, it can lead to various health issues.

One of the most common causes of meridian imbalances is stress. When we experience stress, the body responds by releasing stress hormones that can cause tension and tightness in the muscles, leading to blockages in the meridian system. When these blockages occur, it can lead to a range of physical and emotional symptoms, such as headaches, digestive issues, anxiety, and depression.

To maintain meridian health, there are various practices one can engage in, such as acupuncture, acupressure, and meridian massage. Acupuncture involves the insertion of thin needles into specific points along the meridians to stimulate the flow of qi and promote balance. Acupressure involves applying pressure to these same points to achieve similar effects. Meridian massage is a hands-on therapy that uses pressure and manipulation to stimulate the flow of qi and promote relaxation.

Another way to support meridian health is through a balanced diet. Certain foods are believed to support the health of specific meridians. For example, foods rich in vitamin C, such as citrus fruits, can help support the lung meridian. Similarly, foods rich in omega-3 fatty acids, such as salmon and walnuts, can help support the liver meridian.

Exercise is another crucial component of maintaining meridian health. Exercise helps promote the flow of qi throughout the body, which can help prevent blockages and imbalances. Practices such as yoga, tai chi, and qigong are especially beneficial for promoting meridian health as they focus on movements that support the flow of qi.

In addition to physical practices, emotional and mental health is also essential for maintaining meridian health. Emotions such as anger, fear, and sadness can all contribute to meridian imbalances. Practices such as meditation, mindfulness, and therapy can help promote emotional well-being and prevent meridian imbalances.

Embracing a Meridian-Based Lifestyle for Optimal Well-being

The concept of meridians is central to traditional Chinese medicine (TCM). The twelve major meridians, also known as energy pathways, are believed to carry vital energy, or Qi, throughout the body. These meridians have specific locations and functions, and an imbalance in one or more of them can cause physical or emotional symptoms.

Meridian-based practices, such as acupuncture, acupressure, and meridian massage, have been used for centuries to treat a variety of health issues. However, there is growing interest in the use of meridian-based techniques as a way to promote overall well-being and prevent illness.

Below we will explore the benefits of embracing a meridian-based lifestyle and how it can contribute to optimal health and well-being.

Understanding the Meridian System

The meridian system is a complex network of energy pathways that run throughout the body, connecting different organs and tissues. According to TCM, each meridian is associated with a specific organ or organ system and is responsible for carrying vital energy or Qi to those areas.

The twelve major meridians are:

Lung Meridian

Large Intestine Meridian

Stomach Meridian

Spleen Meridian

Heart Meridian

Small Intestine Meridian

Bladder Meridian

Kidney Meridian

Pericardium Meridian

Triple Warmer Meridian

Gallbladder Meridian

Liver Meridian

Each meridian has a corresponding point on the body that can be stimulated using various techniques to promote the flow of Qi and restore balance to the body.

The Benefits of Meridian-Based Practices

Meridian-based practices, such as acupuncture, acupressure, and meridian massage, have been shown to be effective in treating a variety of health issues. These practices can help alleviate pain, reduce stress, improve sleep, boost immunity, and promote overall well-being.

In addition to treating specific health issues, meridian-based practices can also be used as a preventative measure to maintain overall health and wellness. By promoting the flow of Qi and restoring balance to the body, meridian-based practices can help prevent illness and promote optimal health.

Embracing a Meridian-Based Lifestyle

Incorporating meridian-based practices into your daily routine can help you achieve optimal health and well-being. Here are some tips for embracing a meridian-based lifestyle:

Get regular acupuncture treatments: Acupuncture is a powerful tool for promoting overall health and well-being. Regular acupuncture treatments can help reduce stress, alleviate pain, improve sleep, and boost immunity.

Practice acupressure: Acupressure is a simple yet effective way to promote the flow of Qi and restore balance to the body. You can practice acupressure on yourself or seek the help of a trained professional.

Use essential oils: Essential oils can be used to promote the flow of Qi and support overall well-being. Certain oils, such as lavender and peppermint, have been shown to have a calming effect on the body, while others, such as lemon and grapefruit, can help boost energy levels.

Eat a balanced diet: Eating a balanced diet is essential for maintaining optimal health and well-being. Incorporating foods that support the different meridians can help promote overall health and balance in the body.

Practice mindfulness: Mindfulness practices, such as meditation and yoga, can help reduce stress and promote overall well-being. These practices can also help you become more aware of your body and its needs, making it easier to identify and address imbalances in the meridian system.

Have Questions / Comments?

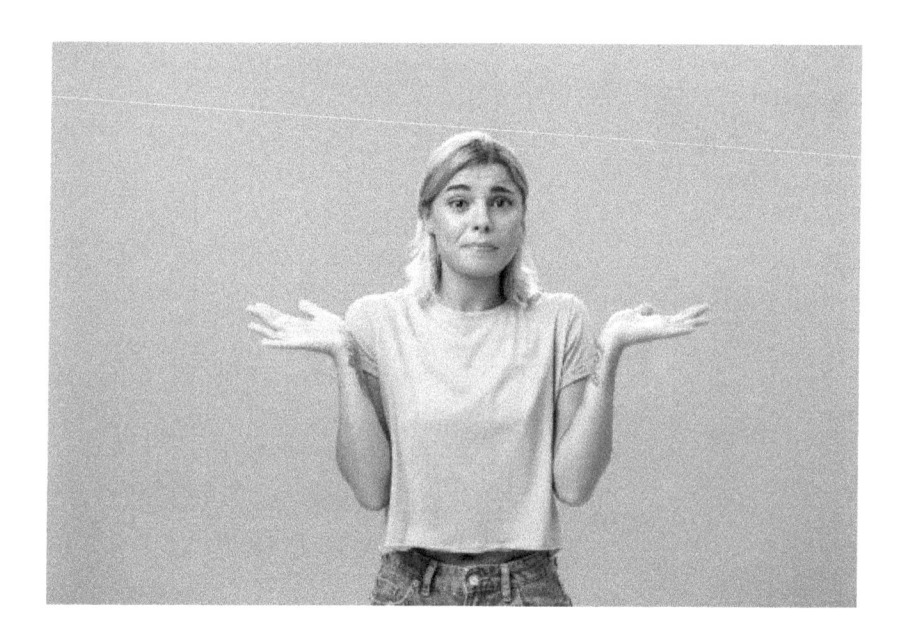

This book was designed to cover as much as possible but I know I have probably missed something, or some new amazing discovery that has just come out.

If you notice something missing or have a question that I failed to answer, please get in touch and let me know. If I can, I will email you an answer and also update the book so others can also benefit from it.

Thanks For Being Awesome :)

Submit Your Questions / Comments At:

https://go.xspurts.com/questions

---

1. https://xspurts.com/posts/questions

Get Another Book Free

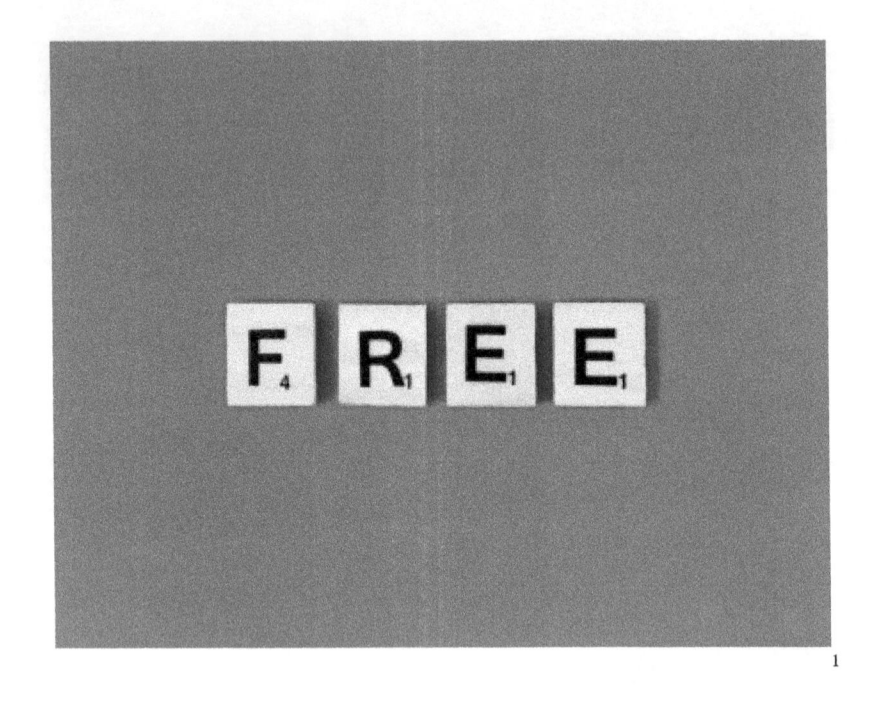

We love writing and have produced a huge number of books.

For being one of our amazing readers, we would love to offer you another book we have created, 100% free.

To claim this limited time special offer, simply go to the site below and enter your name and email address.

You will then receive one of my great books, direct to your email account, 100% free!

https://go.xspurts.com/free-book-offer

---

1. https://xspurts.com/posts/free-book-offer

Also by Mei Lin Zhang

Acupuncture Essentials: Unlocking the Power of Traditional Chinese Medicine
Aromatherapy Unlocked: The Essential Guide to Natural Healing
Demystifying Dit Da: Ancient Wisdom for Modern Healing
Embracing Gua Sha: Traditional Techniques for Modern Living
Feng Shui Fundamentals: Harmonizing Your Space
Moxibustion: Ancient Healing for Modern Living
The Acupressure Handbook: Ancient Healing Techniques for Today's World
The Ayurveda Way Transforming Your Life with Ancient Wisdom
The Meditation Handbook: A Practical Guide to Finding Inner Peace
The Tai Chi Journey: A Path to Mindfulness and Balance
Yin and Yang: Unlocking the Power of Harmony
Chiropractic Unleashed: The Ultimate Guide to Spinal Health
Colon Cleansing: A Path to Optimal Health
Detox Diet Secrets Cleanse, Heal, and Energize Your Body
Ear Candling: A Holistic Approach to Ear Health
Energy Medicine Unlocked: A Comprehensive Guide to Healing
Face Yoga Revolution: Transform Your Skin Naturally
Cupping Therapy Unlocking the Ancient Secrets
Chakra System Mastery: Unlocking Your Inner Power
Destiny and You: An Intertwined Journey
Dopamine Fasting: A Journey to Reclaiming Your Focus and Well-Being
Herbalism Unearthed A Journey Through Nature's Pharmacy

"Hypnosis Unlocked: Mastering the Art of Mind Control "
Jin Shin Do: Unlocking the Body's Healing Power
Johrei: The Power of Divine Energy
Meridian Master A Journey Through the Twelve Major Pathways

Milton Keynes UK
Ingram Content Group UK Ltd.
UKHW020702290124
436892UK00019B/813

9 781776 848683